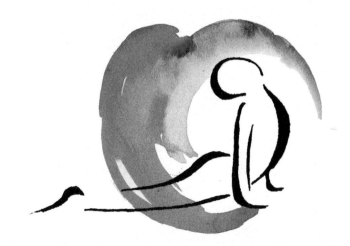

Yogagenda

PLANNER   HANDBOOK   JOURNAL

2016

www.YogagendaS.com

My personal info

_____

_____

_____

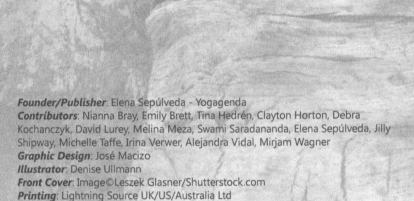

Founder/Publisher: Elena Sepúlveda - Yogagenda
Contributors: Nianna Bray, Emily Brett, Tina Hedrén, Clayton Horton, Debra Kochanczyk, David Lurey, Melina Meza, Swami Saradananda, Elena Sepúlveda, Jilly Shipway, Michelle Taffe, Irina Verwer, Alejandra Vidal, Mirjam Wagner
Graphic Design: José Macizo
Illustrator: Denise Ullmann
Front Cover: Image©Leszek Glasner/Shutterstock.com
Printing: Lightning Source UK/US/Australia Ltd

For more information or to place an order, please visit: www.YogagendaS.com

ISBN: 978-0-9572635-2-9

Disclaimer: The publisher, editor and all contributors disclaim any liability or loss in connection with the theories and practices offered in this *Yogagenda*.

Table
OF CONTENTS

What's IN YOGAGENDA 2016

Namaste and welcome to the fourth edition of *Yogagenda*. Whether you are a returning reader, or this is your first time with us, we are delighted to share with you this ever-evolving yoga publication. This year, our evolving path takes us towards "diversity", because we live yoga through a diversity of choices: it is not only how we practice asana and meditation, but also how we breathe, what our relationship to nature and the wider society is, how we understand health and nutrition, our creative choices, the philosophy behind our actions, how we love as women or men... So be prepared to find a rich diversity of approaches to yoga in this edition! As usual, within this issue you will find *Yogagenda*'s fundamental structure with its three distinctive sections: the **YEARLY PLANNER**, the **YOGA HANDBOOK**, and the **JOURNAL PAGES**.

We hope you enjoy what we are offering you this year. If you have any suggestions, or would like to contribute to future editions of *Yogagenda*, please drop us an email at any time.

And don't forget to visit **www.YogagendaS.com** for: more information about this project; an on-line shop to purchase copies of all *Yogagenda*'s editions; an Inspiration section with book, DVD, film and music suggestions; links to our teacher and healer friends; and all issues of our yoga monthly (-ish) newsletter.

May 2016 be a rich and diverse year for you!

Elena Sepúlveda
Yogagenda Editor
elena@YogagendaS.com

YEARLY PLANNER

We are all about being practical.

This section includes:

⚙ **2 Yearly Calendars** (one for 2016 and another for 2017).

⚙ **1 "Walking the Time Line" double spread.** These pages are an invitation to explore the area of personal responsibility in decision taking. Although time is not necessarily linear and the cause-consequence relationship may be influenced by a myriad of things, it could be helpful to reflect on the decisions you made in 2015, where you are at the moment and the decisions you may need to make in 2016.

⚙ **12 Monthly Calendars**, one per page, with space for notes.

⚙ **52 Week-at-a-Glance Calendars**, with a week on two pages. Weeks are numbered from 1 to 52 and each weekly double spread contains a small **month-at-a-glance calendar, plus information on moon phases, solstices, equinoxes** and **solar/lunar eclipses** for 2016. As we are based in Europe, we have adopted a Northern Hemisphere perspective; if you read us from a different part of the planet, please visit **www.timeanddate.com** for information more relevant to you.

YOGA HANDBOOK

We are all about being informative and, hopefully, inspirational.

As yoga expands and grows in the West, it becomes more and more interdisciplinary. In *Yogagenda*, we enjoy this diversity of approaches that are available to enrich and improve our lives. Reflecting the areas of interest of our contributors, this edition brings together the wisdom of the Vedic and Ayurvedic traditions, of Taoism and Traditional Chinese Medicine, and of Buddhism and meditation. All *Yogagenda* contributors are experts in their fields. Coming from different countries and working all over the world, they are practising yoga teachers, living and breathing within the yogic community worldwide. To find out more about them and their work, please go to **Who Contributed to Yogagenda 2016** (page 236).

This section includes:

⚙ **Six Superfoods with Six Recipes.** Recipes by Irina Verwer and superfoods by Elena Sepúlveda. No symbolism this year, but something much more tangible... and edible! As you move through the different months of the year, you will find a seasonal superfood and an accompanying yummy recipe.

⚙ **Asana Overview**: Yin Asanas for Self-Transformation, by Elena

Sepúlveda. This spread offers suggestions for practising Yin yoga in the context of sthira sukham, as well as the criteria followed for grouping the poses: the five seasons of Traditional Chinese Medicine and their associated elements, meridians/internal organs and emotions.

- **Asana Pages**, illustrated by Denise Ullmann and written by Elena Sepúlveda. There is one Yin asana per month, coded with colours and symbols. Each includes concise instructions on how to get into and exit the pose, a minimum suggested holding time, the meridians and organs it affects, its associated emotions, recommended variations, and its anatomical benefits and contraindications.

- **Superfoods: Natural Choices for Superhealth**. Elena Sepúlveda breaks down the beneficial elements in these nutrient-rich foods and lists some easily available superfoods.

- **Mudras: an Introduction**. Swami Saradananda introduces these powerful hand gestures that are used to stimulate subtle energy in the body.

- **Spring: an Ayurvedic Perspective**. Melina Meza explores the season from the point of view of Ayurveda, the traditional Indian medicine system.

- **Beyond the Mat: Buddhism, Mindful Awareness and Meditation**. Mirjam Wagner reminds us of the need to pause and cultivate awareness in order to allow the benefits of the practice to permeate our daily lives.

- **Home Practice: Sequencing Your Yoga Asanas**. David Lurey offers suggestions to help you create a personal yoga practice that really serves *you*. Please refer to the **Yoga Session Planner** in pp.248-251 to design your own yoga session.

- **Summer: Dancing with Sunlight and Shadow**. Jilly Shipway explores the season in terms of the interplay of light and shadow, offering solstice meditation questions for self-enquiry.

- **Female Power: Yoga and the Divine Feminine**. Nianna Bray celebrates female sexuality and power from a tantric perspective.

- **Conscious Breathing: a Master Key for Health**. Alejandra Vidal encourages us to breathe well and points out the benefits of conscious breathing for our health.

- **Autumn: Life, Yoga and the Body Clock**. Tina Hedrén explores the season from the point of view of Traditional Chinese Medicine and the organs that need looking after during these months.

- **Light on Tapas: Burning Away the Personal Agenda**. Clayton Horton

explains tapas as the work that provides progress and success to any
transformational process.

- ⊚ **Ourmala: Socially Conscious Yoga**.
Emily Brett, founder of Ourmala,
writes about the yoga services
offered to asylum-seekers by this
London-based charity.
- ⊚ **Winter: Yantras, Yoga and You**. Debra Kochanczyk explores the season and introduces us to the world
of mystical diagrams, or yantras.
- ⊚ **Yoga Festivals and Celebrations
around the Globe**. Michelle Taffe
of *The Global Yogi* brings us again
her well-researched listing of yoga
events around the world for 2016.
- ⊚ **Sanskrit Glossary**. These pages
offer short explanations of the Sanskrit terms used in this edition of
Yogagenda.
- ⊚ **Asana Index**. A quick way to find
the Yin poses included in the **Asana
Pages**.
- ⊚ **Yoga Session Planner**. A tem-
plate designed for the purpose of
planning a class or a self-practice
session.
- ⊚ **Patanjali's *Yoga Sutras***. Throughout the weeks you will find the 34
sutras in Sanskrit from the fourth
chapter of Patanjali's *Yoga Sutras*.
Translations into English for these
and the first, second and third
chapters (published in 2012, 2013
and 2014 respectively) can be
found at **www.YogagendaS.com**.

JOURNAL PAGES
*We are all about encouraging creative
reflection.*

This section includes:
- ⊚ Journal or blank pages integrated
at different points in the agenda
(and more at the end too). They
are blank sheets for your own
needs: to do some planning, to
spread your creative wings on
paper, to reflect on the topics
introduced in the articles, or for
whatever takes your fancy.

Walking the 2015–2016 Time Line

2015

at the moment

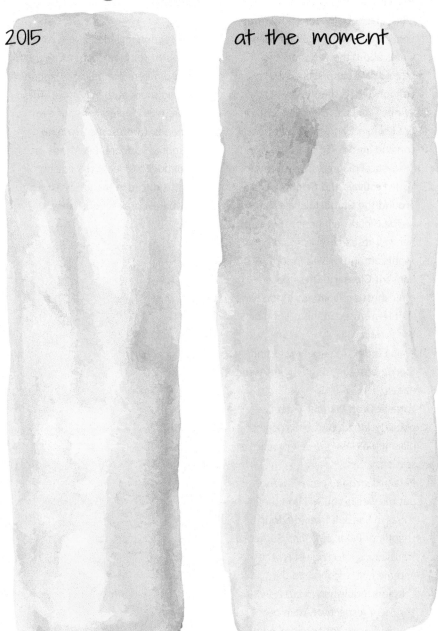

These pages are an invitation to explore the area of personal responsibility in decision taking. Use them to reflect on the decisions you made in 2015, where you are at the moment and the decisions you may need to make in 2016.

2016

2016

January
			1	2	3	
4	5	6	7	8	9	10
11	12	13	14	15	16	17
18	19	20	21	22	23	24
25	26	27	28	29	30	31

February
1	2	3	4	5	6	7
8	9	10	11	12	13	14
15	16	17	18	19	20	21
22	23	24	25	26	27	28
29						

March
	1	2	3	4	5	6
7	8	9	10	11	12	13
14	15	16	17	18	19	20
21	22	23	24	25	26	27
28	29	30	31			

April
				1	2	3
4	5	6	7	8	9	10
11	12	13	14	15	16	17
18	19	20	21	22	23	24
25	26	27	28	29	30	

May
						1
2	3	4	5	6	7	8
9	10	11	12	13	14	15
16	17	18	19	20	21	22
23	24	25	26	27	28	29
30	31					

June
		1	2	3	4	5
6	7	8	9	10	11	12
13	14	15	16	17	18	19
20	21	22	23	24	25	26
27	28	29	30			

July
				1	2	3
4	5	6	7	8	9	10
11	12	13	14	15	16	17
18	19	20	21	22	23	24
25	26	27	28	29	30	31

August
1	2	3	4	5	6	7
8	9	10	11	12	13	14
15	16	17	18	19	20	21
22	23	24	25	26	27	28
29	30	31				

September
			1	2	3	4
5	6	7	8	9	10	11
12	13	14	15	16	17	18
19	20	21	22	23	24	25
26	27	28	29	30		

October
					1	2
3	4	5	6	7	8	9
10	11	12	13	14	15	16
17	18	19	20	21	22	23
24	25	26	27	28	29	30
31						

November
	1	2	3	4	5	6
7	8	9	10	11	12	13
14	15	16	17	18	19	20
21	22	23	24	25	26	27
28	29	30				

December
			1	2	3	4
5	6	7	8	9	10	11
12	13	14	15	16	17	18
19	20	21	22	23	24	25
26	27	28	29	30	31	

2017

January

						1
2	3	4	5	6	7	8
9	10	11	12	13	14	15
16	17	18	19	20	21	22
23	24	25	26	27	28	29
30	31					

February

1	2	3	4	5
6	7	8	9	10	11	12
13	14	15	16	17	18	19
20	21	22	23	24	25	26
27	28					

March

1	2	3	4	5
6	7	8	9	10	11	12
13	14	15	16	17	18	19
20	21	22	23	24	25	26
27	28	29	30	31		

April

					1	2
3	4	5	6	7	8	9
10	11	12	13	14	15	16
17	18	19	20	21	22	23
24	25	26	27	28	29	30

May

1	2	3	4	5	6	7
8	9	10	11	12	13	14
15	16	17	18	19	20	21
22	23	24	25	26	27	28
29	30	31				

June

				1	2	3	4
5	6	7	8	9	10	11
12	13	14	15	16	17	18
19	20	21	22	23	24	25
26	27	28	29	30		

July

					1	2
3	4	5	6	7	8	9
10	11	12	13	14	15	16
17	18	19	20	21	22	23
24	25	26	27	28	29	30
31						

August

1	2	3	4	5	6
7	8	9	10	11	12	13
14	15	16	17	18	19	20
21	22	23	24	25	26	27
28	29	30	31			

September

					1	2	3
4	5	6	7	8	9	10
11	12	13	14	15	16	17
18	19	20	21	22	23	24
25	26	27	28	29	30	

October

						1
2	3	4	5	6	7	8
9	10	11	12	13	14	15
16	17	18	19	20	21	22
23	24	25	26	27	28	29
30	31					

November

1	2	3	4	5
6	7	8	9	10	11	12
13	14	15	16	17	18	19
20	21	22	23	24	25	26
27	28	29	30			

December

				1	2	3
4	5	6	7	8	9	10
11	12	13	14	15	16	17
18	19	20	21	22	23	24
25	26	27	28	29	30	31

January 2016

Monday	Tuesday	Wednesday	Thursday	Friday	Saturday	Sunday
				1	☾ 2	3
4	5	6	7	8	9	○ 10
11	12	13	14	15	16	☽ 17
18	19	20	21	22	23	○ 24
25	26	27	28	29	30	31

February 2016

Monday	Tuesday	Wednesday	Thursday	Friday	Saturday	Sunday
◖ 1	2	3	4	5	6	7
○ 8	9	10	11	12	13	14
◗ 15	16	17	18	19	20	21
○ 22	23	24	25	26	27	28
29						

March 2016

Monday	Tuesday	Wednesday	Thursday	Friday	Saturday	Sunday
		1 ☾ 2	3	4	5	6
7	8 Total Solar Eclipse	○ 9 Total Solar Eclipse	10	11	12	13
14 ☽ 15	16	17	18	19	20 Spring Equinox	
21	22	○ 23	24	25	26	27
28	29	30	☾ 31			

April 2016

Monday	Tuesday	Wednesday	Thursday	Friday	Saturday	Sunday
				1	2	3
4	5	6	○ 7	8	9	10
11	12	13	☽ 14	15	16	17
18	19	20	21	○ 22 Micro Moon	23	24
25	26	27	28	29	☾ 30	

May 2016

Monday	Tuesday	Wednesday	Thursday	Friday	Saturday	Sunday
						1
2	3	4	5	○ 6	7	8
9	10	11	12	☽ 13	14	15
16	17	18	19	20	○ 21 Blue Moon	22
23	24	25	26	27	28	☾ 29
30	31					

June 2016

Monday	Tuesday	Wednesday	Thursday	Friday	Saturday	Sunday
		1	2	3	4	○ 5
6	7	8	9	10	11	☽ 12
13	14	15	16	17	18	19
○ 20	21 Summer Solstice	22	23	24	25	26
☾ 27	28	29	30			

July 2016

Monday	Tuesday	Wednesday	Thursday	Friday	Saturday	Sunday
				1	2	3
● 4	5	6	7	8	9	10
11	☽ 12	13	14	15	16	17
18	19	○ 20	21	22	23	24
25	26	☾ 27	28	29	30	31

August 2016

Monday	Tuesday	Wednesday	Thursday	Friday	Saturday	Sunday
1	○ 2	3	4	5	6	7
8	9	◐ 10	11	12	13	14
15	16	17	○ 18	19	20	21
22	23	24	◑ 25	26	27	28
29	30	31				

September 2016

Monday	Tuesday	Wednesday	Thursday	Friday	Saturday	Sunday
			1 ○ Annular Solar Eclipse	2	3	4
5	6	7	8	9 ☽	10	11
12	13	14	15	16 ○ Penumbal Lunar Eclipse	17	18
19	20	21	22 Autumn Equinox	23 ☾	24	25
26	27	28	29	30		

October 2016

Monday	Tuesday	Wednesday	Thursday	Friday	Saturday	Sunday
					○ 1	2
3	4	5	6	7	8	☽ 9
10	11	12	13	14	15	○ 16
17	18	19	20	21	☾ 22	23
24	25	26	27	28	29	○ 30
31						

November 2016

Monday	Tuesday	Wednesday	Thursday	Friday	Saturday	Sunday
		1	2	3	4	5	6
☾ 7	8	9	10	11	12	13
○ 14 Super Full Moon	15	16	17	18	19	20
☾ 21	22	23	24	25	26	27
28	○ 29	30				

December 2016

Monday	Tuesday	Wednesday	Thursday	Friday	Saturday	Sunday
			1	2	3	4
5	6	☽ 7	8	9	10	11
12	13	○ 14	15	16	17	18
19	20	☾ 21 Winter Solstice	22	23	24	25
26	27	28	○ 29	30	31	

Asana Overview
Yin Asanas for
Self-Transformation

By Elena Sepúlveda

**Paying attention to one particular aspect of asana, sthira sukham, the 12 Yin
asanas featured in this edition of *Yogagenda* aim to serve as a framework
in which to explore the emotional, mental and more spiritual dimensions of
your yoga practice**

STHIRA SUKHAM

Sthira sukham asanam is one of 196 sutras, or aphorisms, found in Patanjali's *Yoga
Sutras* (II.46), the main text of the yogic tradition. Often translated as "posture
must be cultivated with the two qualities of steadiness and ease", it is perhaps
the sutra most frequently quoted in yoga classes. Sthira sukham asanam encourages us to cultivate steadiness and stillness (sthira) in order to find ease (sukham).
But the meaning of the sutra, like the practice of yoga itself, goes well beyond the
edges of our mats or the time slot dedicated to our yoga session.

Bhavani Silvia Maki, in her wonderful book, *The Yogi's Roadmap: The Patanjali Yoga
Sutra as a Journey to Self Realization*, writes: "[Patanjali] recommended the practice
of asana to expand the body's capacity as a container to hold the content within
oneself for examination, and as a leverage to unwind the pattering imprinted in
the nervous system and mind... [He also] emphasised that it is in fact easier to
change the body than the mind, and that deep-seated physiological issues are
best accessed through one's tissues."

So let's start in our bodies: asanas practised cultivating stillness and ease, especially in the face of discomfort, can help us to develop new attitudes and skills; these,
in turn, can prove helpful when facing other types of challenges in our daily lives.

FROM STILLNESS TO EASE THROUGH AWARENESS

Discomfort or tension is felt when stepping outside our familiar comfort zones. However, we all have the capacity to transform that tension into attention or mindful awareness and eventually into ease. In another wonderful book, *Insight Yoga*, Sarah Powers describes mindfulness as "an attitude we adopt in which we let go of all motivations to manipulate the moment and develop the capacity to observe without any wilful interference." This attitude leads to a refined and transformational quality of attention.

The long-held poses of Yin yoga allow time and space for mindful awareness. They provide a context in which to observe the contents of our physical, mental, and emotional bodies, granting us an opportunity for release and self-transformation. As you practice the 12 Yin asanas featured in the *Asana Pages*, you could explore the following:

Begin from where you are...
As always in Yin yoga, come to an appropriate edge at the beginning of each pose. Don't push forward to reach your limits straight away, but allow time for the body to adjust and perhaps go further after a few rounds of breaths, when you feel the tissues giving up their first resistance.

Connect with your breath...
Tune into your breath to cultivate concentration. Even out the inhalation and the exhalation, counting to 5 or 6 each time. Deepening and slowing the breath soothes the nervous system and invites the mind to calm down and focus. To learn more about the connection between breath and mind, read our article on *Conscious Breathing* by Alejandra Vidal (pp.146-149).

Pay close attention to your physical sensations...
Observe any physical tensions. Be willing to experience the moment and become aware of any subtle changes as you spend time in the pose. Remember that where attention goes, vital energy (and ease) flows! But be wise and lessen the intensity if you feel you could be stepping into harm.

Practice surrendering...
Hold your attention without judging and especially let go of any strategies of evasion, avoidance, denial or struggle.

Become aware of your thoughts and/or emotions...

Thoughts or emotions may arise to the forefront of your awareness. Give them the same treatment: stay present and non-reactive. Being connected without react-ing allows you to experience them as less solid and threatening; to view them with some detachment rather than being over-identified with them ("I'm feeling anger or fear" instead of "I'm angry or fearful").

Notice them change...

In the same way that body sensations transform themselves as time unfolds in the pose and vital energy flows into the areas of discomfort, emotions and thoughts also change. They may lessen in intensity, or even disappear with time. At some point, try to move your focus of attention from the emotion or thought itself to your aversion of it—or craving for others.

Ultimately, these two movements of the mind, craving and aversion, are partly responsible for our being stuck in duhkha, or suffering, instead of the opposite, sukha, or ease.

The sutra sthira sukham asanam encourages us to adopt this attitude in every-thing we do, not just asana practice. To explore further this aspect, please read our article on *Buddhism, Mindful Awareness and Meditation* by Mirjam Wagner (pp.78-80).

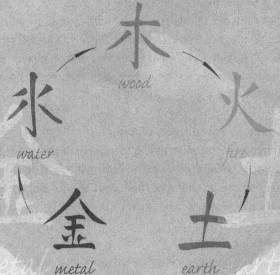

YIN ASANAS AND EMOTIONS

Yin yoga is based on Traditional Chinese Medicine, in which the cycle of life has five seasons associated with five elements and five main emotions. Each season's element is also associated with two complementary internal organs connected by a network of meridians, or energetic paths. Yin asanas help harmonise the flow of energy along the meridians, bringing health to internal organs and balancing their associated emotions. Asanas have been grouped here by season, element, emotion and meridian/internal organ.

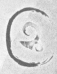

Winter – Water – Fear / Wisdom
Half Butterfly and the Urinary Bladder meridian (pp.44-45)
Deer and the Kidney meridian (pp.60-61)
Dangling and the Urinary Bladder meridian (pp.228-229)

Spring – Wood – Anger / Compassion
Frog and the Liver meridian (pp.78-79)
Shoelace and the Gall Bladder meridian (pp.94-95)
Sleeping Swan and the Gall Bladder meridian (pp.110-111)

Summer – Fire – Hate / Love
Seal and the Heart / Small Intestine meridians (pp.128-129)
Shoulder Stretch and the Heart meridian (pp.144-145)

Late Summer – Earth – Anxiety / Calmness
Dragon Flying Low and the Stomach meridian (pp.160-161)
Half Saddle Variation and the Spleen meridian (pp.178-179)

Autumn – Metal – Sadness / Courage
Caterpillar and the Lung meridian (pp.194-195)
Cat Pulling its Tail and the Large Intestine meridian (pp.210-211)

NOTE: Please bear in mind that not all yoga poses and variations are suitable for all people. It is your responsibility to know your body and its limitations and to choose a practice that is appropriate for you.

SuperFoods:

Natural Choices for Superhealth

By Elena Sepúlveda

Sometimes exotic, sometimes easily found in your local market or grocery store, superfoods are nutrient- or phytochemical- rich edibles with numerous health and well-being benefits. Including them in our diets will expose us to a world of goodness

Superfoods are natural powerhouses of proteins, essential amino acids, vitamins, minerals, antioxidants, essential fatty acids and fibre. Since all these work together as a "team", it is in our best interest to respect the innate wisdom of nature and obtain them from fresh foods (fruits, vegetables, legumes, grains, nuts, seeds, etc.), rather than as isolated and synthesised elements. Here is a little insight into each one of these elements.

PROTEINS build, maintain, and replace body tissues such as cells, muscles, organs, connective tissue, bones, neurotransmitters, genes, etc. They are made up of many types of amino acids, although 22 of them are crucial. Of these, 13 can be produced by the body itself and the other nine can only be obtained from protein-rich foods.

ESSENTIAL AMINO ACIDS, the building blocks of proteins, are those nine amino acids we can only get from food. They are available to any-one who consumes a wide variety of vegetarian foods.

VITAMINS are organic compounds needed for normal body growth and functions. Since our body cannot produce enough of these on its own, it gets them in very small amounts from the food we eat. How much of these vitamins will end up in our blood depends on our digestive ability, therefore it is important to make sure our digestive system is clean and not overtaxed.

MINERALS are inorganic substances found in the earth's soils and rocks. For the human body to be able to use them, they need to be part of the structure of plants. Plants do not synthesize minerals (unlike vitamins); instead they take up mineral salts from the soil and convert them into colloidal minerals (organic compounds) which can then be then absorbed by the body.

ANTIOXIDANTS prevent or slow down the oxidative damage caused by free radicals, the by-product naturally generated when the cells use oxygen to transfer the energy stored in food into a usable form. Wholesome foods will automatically self-regulate free radical activity, since the antioxidants they contain are biochemically balanced in terms of anti- and pro-oxidants.

ESSENTIAL FATTY ACIDS are the crucial building blocks of fat (fuel!) in our body. The human body needs fat for many functions, from regulating thyroid and adrenal activity or blood pressure to maintaining brain and nerve function. The two main fatty acids we need to include in our diet so they can be absorbed into the blood are Omega 3 and Omega 6 (our body can't synthesise them itself).

FIBRE consists of carbohydrates that cannot be digested; consequently, their sugar units are not absorbed into the bloodstream. They help food move through our digestive system, feed the "good bacteria" that make vitamin B12 and release fatty acids, and regulate bowel action.

As with everything we eat or drink, superfoods are richest in nutrients and exercise their healing properties best when they are organic (without pesticides, fresher, better for the environment, and GMO-free) and their processing is healthy (additive and preservative free).

Vegan foodie and yoga teacher Irina Verwer has contributed to *Yogagenda*

2016 six delicious recipes for six powerful superfoods. You'll find them at the beginning of each month: first the superfood, then the recipe the following month. In addition, other easily available superfood suggestions can be found below. For more scrumptious recipes, check her site **IrinaVerwer.com**.

Here are some favourite superfoods:

Almonds: rich in protein, fibre, calcium and magnesium.

Avocados: contain glutathione, a powerful antioxidant.

Asparagus: rich in vitamin K, but also a natural diuretic that can alleviate bloating.

Beetroots: with a unique combination of phytochemicals and minerals, they can help fight infections, purify the blood and cleanse the liver.

Brazil nuts: extremely rich in selenium.

Cabbages: with antibacterial and antiviral properties, they help the liver break down excess hormones and cleanse the digestive tract.

Cranberries: also have antibacterial and antiviral properties, and they help cleanse the urinary tract.

Flaxseeds: very rich in essential fatty acids, especially Omega 3.

Garlic: another powerful antibacterial

that helps lower blood pressure by cleansing build-up from the arteries; it also helps cleanse the respiratory tract, expelling mucus built up in lungs and sinuses.

"As with everything we eat or drink, superfoods are richest in nutrients and exercise their healing properties best when they are organic (without pesticides, fresher, better for the environment, and GMO-free) and their processing is healthy (additive and preservative free)."

Lemons: with more than 20 anti-cancer compounds and plenty of vitamin C, they help keep the body alkaline.

Seaweeds: Loaded with minerals and trace minerals, they bind to radioactive waste and heavy metals in the body so they can be removed.

Sun-dried plums: packed with a phytochemical called polyphenol that boosts bone density by stimulating bone-building cells.

Sunflower seeds: very rich in vitamin E.

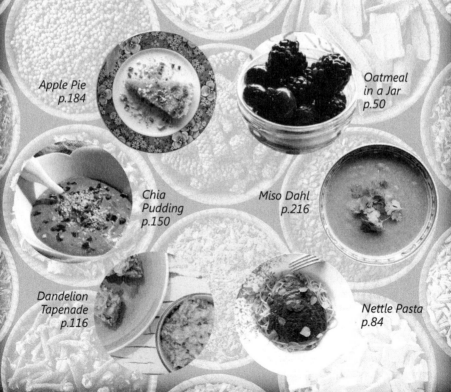

Apple Pie
p.184

Oatmeal
in a Jar
p.50

Chia
Pudding
p.150

Miso Dahl
p.216

Dandelion
Tapenade
p.116

Nettle Pasta
p.84

my notes

_____

_____

_____

_____

_____

_____

_____

_____

_____

_____

_____

_____

_____

_____

_____

_____

_____

_____

_____

_____

_____

_____

_____

_____

OATS: The Ultimate Winter Breakfast

Oats have been cultivated in many places and consumed as food, as well as used for medicinal purposes, for at least two thousand years. Harvested in autumn and available all year round, we could consider them to be the ultimate winter breakfast to keep us fuelled up. Oats may not look very impressive, but they do have an impressive nutritional profile. They are rich in beta-glucans, a type of soluble fibre with numerous benefits, such as inhibiting the body's absorption of bad cholesterol; slowing down the absorption of carbohydrates into the blood stream and therefore avoiding spikes of sugar blood and insulin levels; or boosting the immune system against bacteria, viruses, fungi and parasites. Oats also provide plenty of magnesium, which helps to prevent heart problems by relaxing blood vessels, aiding the heart muscle and regulating blood pressure.

January 2016

January 2016

				1	2	3
4	5	6	7	8	9	10
11	12	13	14	15	16	17
18	19	20	21	22	23	24
25	26	27	28	29	30	31

28
MONDAY

29
TUESDAY

30
WEDNESDAY

Patanjali's Yoga Sutras – Chapter IV: Kaivalya Pada

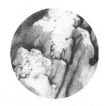

31
THURSDAY

1
FRIDAY

Last Quarter 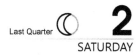 **2**
SATURDAY

3
SUNDAY

January 2016

				1	2	3	week 53
4	5	6	7	8	9	10	
11	12	13	14	15	16	17	
18	19	20	21	22	23	24	
25	26	27	28	29	30	31	

January 2016

4
MONDAY

5
TUESDAY

6
WEDNESDAY

Sutra IV.1 *janmausadhi mantra tapah samadhi jah siddhayah*

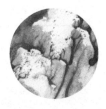

7
THURSDAY

8
FRIDAY

9
SATURDAY

New Moon ○ **10**
SUNDAY

January 2016

			1	2	3
4	5	6	7	8	9	10
11	12	13	14	15	16	17
18	19	20	21	22	23	24
25	26	27	28	29	30	31

week 1

11
MONDAY

12
TUESDAY

13
WEDNESDAY

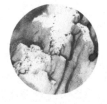

14
THURSDAY

15
FRIDAY

16
SATURDAY

First Quarter

17
SUNDAY

January 2016

				1	2	3
4	5	6	7	8	9	10
11	12	13	14	15	16	17	week 2
18	19	20	21	22	23	24
25	26	27	28	29	30	31

January 2016

18
MONDAY

19
TUESDAY

20
WEDNESDAY

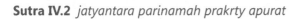

Sutra IV.2 *jatyantara parinamah prakrty apurat*

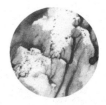

January 2016

21
THURSDAY

22
FRIDAY

23
SATURDAY

Full Moon ○ **24**
SUNDAY

January 2016

				1	2	3
4	5	6	7	8	9	10
11	12	13	14	15	16	17
18	19	20	21	22	23	24
25	26	27	28	29	30	31

week 3

January 2016

25
MONDAY

26
TUESDAY

27
WEDNESDAY

Sutra IV.3 *nimittam aprayojakam prakrtinam varanabhedas tu tatah ksetrikavat*

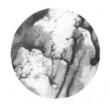

28
THURSDAY

29
FRIDAY

30
SATURDAY

31
SUNDAY

January 2016

				1	2	3
4	5	6	7	8	9	10
11	12	13	14	15	16	17
18	19	20	21	22	23	24
25	26	27	28	29	30	31

week 4

Half Butterfly
Winter - Water - Fear / Wisdom

Start from a comfortable sitting position with both legs stretched

Bring the right foot towards your pelvis while keeping the left one extended

Place your hands on the floor to either side of your left leg

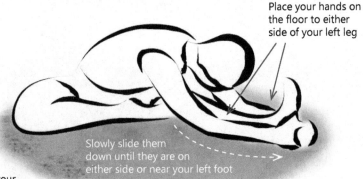

Slowly slide them down until they are on either side or near your left foot

Allow your back and head to relax without engaging your neck, arm or leg muscles

While in the Pose

- Holding time: at least 3 minutes on each side.
- Explore suggestions in pp.25-26.

Coming out of the Pose

- Leave the pose slowly and mindfully.
- Inhale and gradually come back to an upright position. Stretch your right leg forward. Place your hands on the ground behind your hips with your arms extended and rest back creating a very mild back bend. Repeat on the other side.
- Observe the effects of the pose.

Modifications and Variations

- If you suffer from a pulled hamstring, place a cushion under your extended knee so there is no full extension in the leg.
- Rest your bent knee on a cushion or move that foot way from you if you feel any pain in the knee.

Taking it Further

- Take back the foot of the bent leg into Half Virasana (Hero Pose). This will help the hip to fold further forward, but make sure it is safe for your knee.

Meridian and Associated Emotions

This pose stimulates the Urinary Bladder meridian as it flows through either side of the spine and down into the back of the legs, bringing health to this internal organ. The emotions associated with it are Fear (imbalanced) and Wisdom (balanced).

Anatomical Benefits

It stretches the lower back.
It stimulates the ligaments along the back of the spine.

Contraindications

Sciatica.
Knee issues.
Pulled hamstrings.

my notes

Mudras:
an Introduction

By Swami Saradananda

Studied by yogis for millennia, these powerful hand gestures are used to channel and stimulate subtle energy within the body. They can be combined with other exercises, as is the case here of Nadānusandhana and the chanting of the sacred sound OM

Before human beings used spoken language, we used our hands and bodily gestures to communicate. Although speaking with your hands is frequently seen as undignified in modern life in some cultures, no part of your body, aside from your face, expresses your emotions as much. Your hands, with their ability to make a wide range of gestures and subtle movements, help you to convey your thoughts and feelings. How your fingers move and touch each other influences the flow of subtle energy within your body. Modern science has found that the way you move your hands and fingers influences which portions of your brain are activated.

For thousands of years, yogis have researched and used precise hand and finger gestures, known as mudras, to channel prana (subtle energy). They found that many of these movements promoted physical and mental healing; others helped them to expand consciousness.

Mudra is the Sanskrit word for "seal". By working with these gestures, you are sealing and focusing your subtle energy. There are probably thousands of different mudras; many are extremely functional, simple to perform, safe and effective. Although the shape and flexibility of your fingers might influence how easily you can come into a mudra, with practice the increased flexibility that you gain will overcome the initial obstacles.

When performing a mudra, a light contact between your thumb and other finger(s) is sufficient; strong pressure is not really required. Unless otherwise specified, it is usually best to do mudras with both hands simultaneously.

Mudras stimulate your subtle energy and also help you to achieve harmony on both an individual and universal level. Many of their benefits are enhanced by doing them in conjunction with other exercises, such as meditation, visualisation, pranayama, mantra chanting and *asana* practice.

NADĀNUSANDHANA: FOUR-PART MUDRA SERIES WITH OM

Nadānusandhana is a four-part series of mudras practised alongside the different sounds that make up the mantra **OM**. First you chant the component parts **A**, **U** and **M** while practising three mudras, and then you chant the full mantra itself while holding the final mudra.

In yoga philosophy, **OM** is the sound of the infinite, representing all that was, is and shall be. The **A** sound represents the past, waking and the physical plane, the **OU** sound the present, dreaming and the mental plane, while the **M** sound stands for the future, deep sleep and everything beyond comprehension by the mind and intellect. The silence that comes after you finish chanting deepens your inner awareness and releases any subtle tensions that might be present in your mind.

1 Chin Mudra while chanting 'AAAA'

Come into a sitting position. Bring your hands into Chin Mudra by joining the tips of your thumbs and index fingers. Keep the other fingers straight, but relaxed. Rest the backs of your hands on your thighs. Open your mouth wide and inhale deeply. Keeping your mouth wide open, exhale slowly as you chant an elongated '**AAAA**'. Repeat this nine times, feeling the sound resonating in your abdomen.

2 Chinmaya Mudra while chanting 'OU'

Keep your thumbs and index fingers joined; bend the middle, ring and little fingers on each hand until they touch their respective palms. Rest the backs of your hands on your thighs. Inhale deeply, open your mouth halfway and round your lips. As you exhale, chant an elongated '**OU**'. Repeat this nine times, noticing the sound resonating in your chest and throat regions.

3 Adi Mudra while chanting 'MMMM'

Make fists with the thumbs inside your fingers. Rest the backs of your hands on your thighs. Keeping your lips gently together, breathe in through your nose. As you exhale, chant an elongated '**MMMM**'. Repeat this nine times, feeling the sound vibrating in your head and face.

"Mudras stimulate your subtle energy and also help you to achieve harmony on both an individual and universal level. Many of their benefits are enhanced by doing them in conjunction with other exercises, such as meditation, visualisation, pranayama, mantra chanting and asana practice."

4 Brahma Mudra while chanting 'AUM'

Place your fists on either side of your navel. Inhale deeply and open your mouth wide. As you exhale, chant '**A-U-M**'. Feel your mouth gradually rounding until your lips are completely together. Repeat this nine times, feeling the sound resonating throughout your body.

my notes

_____
_____
_____
_____
_____
_____
_____
_____
_____
_____
_____
_____
_____
_____
_____
_____
_____
_____
_____
_____
_____
_____
_____
_____
_____
_____

OATMEAL IN A JAR

Here is a basic recipe, but feel free to experiment, especially with toppings; the possibilities are literally endless!

- *1/3 cup oats*
- *2 tbs chia seeds*
- *Cinnamon, nutmeg, vanilla and/or ginger to taste*

- *1 cup water, rice milk, coconut milk or almond milk*
- *Toppings: 1 tbs nut butter or coconut oil, a handful of fresh or dried fruits, avocado, cacao nibs...*

Put the oats, chia seeds and spices in a jar. Shake and take with you wherever you go. Add the liquid at least thirty minutes before you wish to eat your oatmeal. Shake, wait and top with whatever toppings you prefer. When you are on the road, you can also add the toppings to the dry mixture and let them soak as well. Raisins, dates, nuts and cacao nibs work very well. Just remember that you need to add an extra splash of liquid with them.

February 2016

February 2016

1	2	3	4	5	6	7
8	9	10	11	12	13	14
15	16	17	18	19	20	21
22	23	24	25	26	27	28
29						

February 2016

1
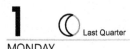 Last Quarter
MONDAY

2
TUESDAY

3
WEDNESDAY

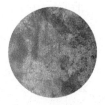

February 2016

4
THURSDAY

5
FRIDAY

6
SATURDAY

7
SUNDAY

February 2016

1	2	3	4	5	6	7	week 5
8	9	10	11	12	13	14	
15	16	17	18	19	20	21	
22	23	24	25	26	27	28	
29							

February 2016

8
New Moon

MONDAY

9
TUESDAY

10
WEDNESDAY

Sutra IV.4 *nirmana cittany asmita matrat*

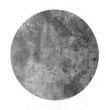

11
THURSDAY

12
FRIDAY

13
SATURDAY

14
SUNDAY

February 2016

1	2	3	4	5	6	7
8	9	10	11	12	13	14	week 6
15	16	17	18	19	20	21
22	23	24	25	26	27	28
29						

15 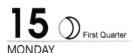 First Quarter
MONDAY

16
TUESDAY

17
WEDNESDAY

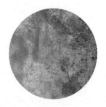

Sutra IV.5 *pravrtti bhede prayojakam cittam ekam anekesam*

18
THURSDAY

19
FRIDAY

20
SATURDAY

21
SUNDAY

February 2016

1	2	3	4	5	6	7
8	9	10	11	12	13	14
15	16	17	18	19	20	21
22	23	24	25	26	27	28
29						

week 7

February 2016

22
○ Full Moon
MONDAY

23
TUESDAY

24
WEDNESDAY

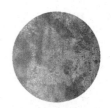

25
THURSDAY

26
FRIDAY

27
SATURDAY

28
SUNDAY

February 2016

1	2	3	4	5	6	7
8	9	10	11	12	13	14
15	16	17	18	19	20	21
22	23	24	25	26	27	28

week 8

29

Deer

Winter - Water - Fear / Wisdom

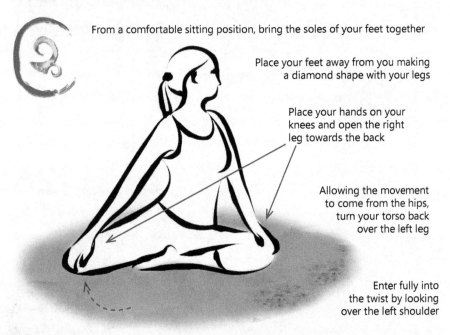

From a comfortable sitting position, bring the soles of your feet together

Place your feet away from you making a diamond shape with your legs

Place your hands on your knees and open the right leg towards the back

Allowing the movement to come from the hips, turn your torso back over the left leg

Enter fully into the twist by looking over the left shoulder

While in the Pose

- Holding time: at least 1 minute on each side.
- Explore suggestions in pp.25-26.

Coming out of the Pose

- Leave the pose slowly and mindfully.
- Exhale, turn your torso to the front and gently twist in the opposite direction, allowing the movement to start again from the hips. Repeat on the other side.
- Observe the effects of the pose.

Modifications and Variations

- To make sure both sitting bones are on the floor, move both feet closer to your body.
- Place a cushion or blanket under to your front knee to protect it, or under the opposite buttock so you don't tilt too much to one side.

Taking it Further

- Move both feet away from your hips to increase the stretch in the inner legs.
- Twist further past the front leg and rest on your elbows or bring your head to the floor.

Meridian and Associated Emotions

This pose stimulates the Kidney meridian as it flows up through the inside of both legs and through the lumbar area, bringing health to these internal organs. The emotions associated with them are Fear (imbalanced) and Wisdom (balanced).

Anatomical Benefits

It provides a balanced internal and external rotation of the hips.
It stretches the groins and the IT band (exterior upper leg).

Contraindications

Knee issues.

my notes

SPRING:
an Ayurvedic
Perspective

By Melina Meza

As spring dawns in our lives and we enter the most energetic and creative time of the year, this article explores the season from the point of view of Ayurveda, the traditional Indian medicine system that uses the principles of nature to maintain health and balance

Since we are part of nature, we have the opportunity to be graceful and let the seasons flow without clinging or grasping. It is natural to have preferences for certain seasons, times of year that resonate with our core elements and make us feel more like ourselves. And yet, developing equanimity and contentment with all seasons -regardless of dosha, or where you live- is essential to well-being. This is where the art of sequencing can be instrumental and of great benefit.

Envision a comma -a momentary pause, after each season- no matter where you live. Your body can benefit from experiencing and adapting to new environments, exercise routines, and foods. It will grow stronger, be more resilient, and keep you in touch with the cycles of nature. The yogis believe that you are one with nature and that in order for you to bloom, you need diversity.

Spring is the most dynamic, energetic and creative time of the year. Nature wakes up from her resting phase full of vitality, which she uses to manifest her creative vision after a long sleep. With sufficient rest in the wintertime, you, too, should feel the "spring fever" or "pulse" that pushes you to stretch or be physical, cleanse, start creative projects, or sow new seeds and intentions that will broaden your horizon in the near future.

In Ayurveda, spring is all about the kapha (water/earth elements) dosha releasing into a pitta (fire/water elements) phase. Doshas occurs when our natural state of health is out of whack, often due to improper eating, overuse of our senses, not enough sleep, or misalignment with the seasons. From the Ayurvedic perspective, when the earth element is balanced, a person will typically have a stable constitution, good stamina, and a strong mind that does not fatigue easily. As soon as there is sufficient solar heat to soften and melt the frozen earth, notice where the changes in your own body fluids are taking place.

In nature you will see fast-moving rivers, perhaps even floods, at the same time that your body is more susceptible to runny noses, chest colds, or excess mucus.

One of my favourite nutritionists, Elson Hass, M.D., said, "Elimination equals illumination," which is a good mantra for this time of the year. I often recommend to students and clients that their spring ritual begin by cleaning their house, refrigerator, and closet, places that often store items we no longer use or that have reached their expiration date. Cleansing your body is a lot like cleaning your house. If you never cleaned your house, it would be difficult to move around the piles lurking in every corner.

A similar thing happens in your digestive tract, especially if you are not consuming enough fibre or hydrating liquids. Blocked channels in the body become breeding grounds for disease and parasites as partially digested food matter putrefies in congested places in the GI tract or elsewhere. Our body, just like nature, needs space. The lack of space in the digestive channels eventually leads to slower movement of food down the GI tract and decreased absorption of the essential nutrients from the food we eat. In Ayurveda, we believe that protecting your digestive fire is the most important factor in maintaining your physical and mental health!

If your organs are not cleansed with twisting yoga poses or pressed into with forward bends, they, too, can build up a film or sludge around the organs that obstructs subtle energy flow and decreases efficiency. By taking a little extra time in the spring season for internal cleansing, your body will reward you tenfold as it starts to run more efficiently. The payoff will be more energy to do everything you love.

"Cleansing your body is a lot like cleaning your house. If you never cleaned your house, it would be difficult to move around the piles lurking in every corner. A similar thing happens in your digestive tract, especially if you are not consuming enough fibre or hydrating liquids."

my notes

_____
_____
_____
_____
_____
_____
_____
_____
_____
_____
_____
_____
_____
_____
_____
_____
_____
_____
_____
_____
_____
_____
_____
_____
_____
_____

NETTLE: Wild and Wonderful

Better known for its medicinal properties when drunk as tea, this stinging wild plant is highly nutritious and can be used in soups or cooked like any other leafy vegetable. Its tender stems, gathered in spring before they flower, are delicious simply steamed and seasoned with butter and lemon. Incorporating nettle into our diets will provide a huge boost in vitamin A, including vitamin A as beta-carotene, which is a key to good vision and strong immunity. Nettle is also a good source of vitamin C, iron, and calcium, while dried nettle is high in protein. Easy-to-absorb amino acids, the building blocks of proteins and essential for healing wounds and repairing tissue, are also found abundantly in this plant. Eating nettle is said to relieve seasonal allergies and to promote healthy adrenal glands and kidneys by encouraging the body to expel toxins (detoxifying).

March 2016

March 2016

	1	2	3	4	5	6
7	8	9	10	11	12	13
14	15	16	17	18	19	20
21	22	23	24	25	26	27
28	29	30	31			

29
MONDAY

1
TUESDAY

2
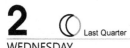 Last Quarter
WEDNESDAY

Sutra IV.6 *tatra dhyanajam anasayam*

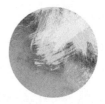

3
THURSDAY

4
FRIDAY

5
SATURDAY

6
SUNDAY

March 2016

	1	2	3	4	5	6	week 9
7	8	9	10	11	12	13	
14	15	16	17	18	19	20	
21	22	23	24	25	26	27	
28	29	30	31				

March 2016

7
MONDAY

8
TUESDAY   Total Solar Eclipse

9
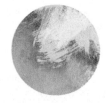 New Moon

WEDNESDAY   Total Solar Eclipse

Sutra IV.7 *karmasuklakrsnam yoginas trividham itaresam*

10
THURSDAY

11
FRIDAY

12
SATURDAY

13
SUNDAY

March 2016

	1	2	3	4	5	6	
7	8	9	10	11	12	13	week 10
14	15	16	17	18	19	20	
21	22	23	24	25	26	27	
28	29	30	31				

March 2016

14
MONDAY

15 ◗ First Quarter
TUESDAY

16
WEDNESDAY

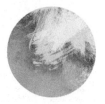

17
THURSDAY

18
FRIDAY

19
SATURDAY

20
Spring Equinox   SUNDAY

March 2016

1	2	3	4	5	6	
7	8	9	10	11	12	13
14	15	16	17	18	19	20	week 11
21	22	23	24	25	26	27
28	29	30	31			

21
MONDAY

22
TUESDAY

23 ○ Full Moon
WEDNESDAY

Sutra IV.8 *tatas tadvipakanugunanam evabhivyaktir vasananam*

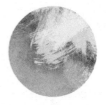

24
THURSDAY

25
FRIDAY

26
SATURDAY

27
SUNDAY

March 2016

	1	2	3	4	5	6
7	8	9	10	11	12	13
14	15	16	17	18	19	20
21	22	23	24	25	26	27
28	29	30	31			

week 12

28
MONDAY

29
TUESDAY

30
WEDNESDAY

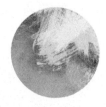

Sutra IV.9 *jati desa kala vyavahitanam apy anantaryam smrti samskarayor ekarupatvat*

Last Quarter ☽ **31**
THURSDAY

1
FRIDAY

2
SATURDAY

3
SUNDAY

March 2016

	1	2	3	4	5	6
7	8	9	10	11	12	13
14	15	16	17	18	19	20
21	22	23	24	25	26	27
28	29	30	31			

week 13

Frog
Spring - Wood - Anger / Compassion

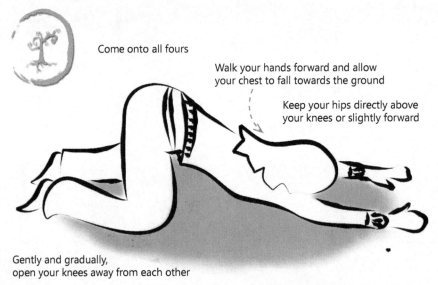

Come onto all fours

Walk your hands forward and allow your chest to fall towards the ground

Keep your hips directly above your knees or slightly forward

Gently and gradually, open your knees away from each other

Let your heart melt towards the ground

While in the Pose
- Holding time: at least 3 minutes.
- Explore suggestions in pp.25-26.

Coming out of the Pose
- Leave the pose slowly and mindfully.
- Inhale, walk with your hands towards you, and lift your torso to come onto all fours again. Bring your knees closer and sit back on your heels in Balasana (Child's Pose).
- Observe the effects of the pose.

Modifications and Variations
- If you feel a painful pressure in the neck, rest one cheek on the ground and change to the other side halfway into the pose.
- Sit back on your heels if you feel too much pressure on the lower back.
- Place some padding under your knees if necessary.

Taking it Further
- Put your feet in flex and separate them until they are in line with your knees (right behind them and creating a 90 degrees angle).
- Place your chin on the floor instead of your forehead or cheek.

Meridian and Associated Emotions

This pose stimulates the Liver meridian as it flows up through the inside of the legs, bringing health to this internal organ. The emotions associated with it are Anger (imbalanced) and Compassion (balanced).

Anatomical Benefits

It stretches the groins and adductor muscles.
It applies healthy stress on the lower back.
It opens up the throat, shoulders, armpits, chest, and belly when arms are stretched and the chin is on the floor.

Contraindications

Lower back injuries.
Knee issues.
Neck tension.

my notes

Beyond the Mat:
Buddhism,
Mindful Awareness
and Meditation

By Mirjam Wagner

Both the Buddhist and the yogic traditions remind us in their own ways that we need to stop, become still, and cultivate awareness to allow the benefits of our practice to permeate and transform our daily lives

STHIRA SUKHAM ASANAM

This principle of the yogic tradition reminds practitioners not to lose themselves in the effort of achieving a pose but always to look for *stability and comfort*, no matter what pose they are in. The tight, concentrated faces and contracted bodies we often see in a yoga class prove that this is not as simple as it sounds, whether on the yoga mat or out in real life.

"PAUSE, SOFTEN, CONNECT"

With these three simple words, Sarah Powers, my beloved teacher and mentor, opens all of her sessions, whether she is guiding through a deep meditation or giving one of her insightful and nourishing lectures about Buddhism and mindful awareness. *Pause, soften, connect* is a warm, well-deserved invitation to the core of our hearts to stop striving, fixing or improving. Everyone who has ever followed this simple instruction knows the immediate relief and healing effect of it. When we invite stability and comfort (sthira sukham), we make space for our souls to arise to the surface.

The ancient teachings of Buddhism also offer us wonderful keys for bringing comfort and stability into our daily lives, both physically and mentally, whether we are heading towards work in a crowded metro station, handling the challenging schedule of family life, or dealing with demanding customers who stress our nervous systems to their highest level.

"LEAVE EVERYTHING AS IT IS AND REST YOUR WEARY MIND"

This is one of the important messages from Buddhism that brings peace of mind and influences our whole being in a positive way: jaw and shoulder muscles relax, breath and vital energy flow freely through our systems, and solutions for daily problems are easier to find.

However, these words may also provoke a sensation of aversion and anger in the Western population: "How do you think I will get my bills paid, my children fed, and my job done if I let go of fighting my way through all my worldly obligations? Problems do not disappear by themselves!"

These points are valid, yet they ignore the fact that constant worrying and a rigid attitude are not helpful for going through life in a healthy and successful way. The more we tighten and the more uncomfortable we get, the more we lose our inner stability and the connection to ourselves.

Instead, if we let go of constant worrying and start to breathe fully and in a relaxed manner, we allow energy and creativity to flow freely through the body, our minds work with clarity and efficiency, and our souls can continue their natural healing process.

There are three powerful tools for practising sthira sukham in our daily lives:

1. Mindful Awareness

If we want to heal ourselves, we need to know ourselves.

If we want to know ourselves, we need to listen and look deeper. Self-observation is one of the most accessible yet challenging tasks to integrate into our lives. Only if we practise mindful awareness are we able to make necessary changes when feeling unsteady or uncomfortable.

2. Meditation
Look for stillness! Train the body and mind to be still at least once a day. As the world we live in does not make it easy to relax and open up, start in places where you feel safe: at home, in nature, and in meditation centres, churches or other spiritual places. Start with 20 minutes a day and choose a quiet time to be steady and comfortable in body and mind.

3. Inner Attitude
We have a choice as to where we focus our attention.
We can decide what our priorities are in life and we can use our minds to relax body, breath and thoughts.

It is very uplifting to see students come out from a workshop, retreat or training with this powerful and peaceful state of mind combined with a relaxed and healthy body. However, many struggle to maintain this attitude while back in busy and competitive worlds. It is not easy to give up a mentality of constant alert

"Pause, soften, connect is a warm, well-deserved invitation to the core of our hearts to stop striving, fixing or improving. Everyone who has ever followed this simple instruction knows the immediate relief and healing effect of it. When we invite stability and comfort (sthira sukham), we make space for our souls to arise to the surface."

and physical tension when fear of losing job, status, or even family is present.

Remember that everything new needs to be trained and requires patience! It only takes a reminder to breathe, a moment to be still and the decision to pause, soften, and connect and let sthira sukham become part of our nature.

To explore this aspect of sthira sukham in asana practice further, please read the *Asana Overview* pages (pp.24-27).

my notes

_____

_____

_____

_____

_____

_____

_____

_____

_____

_____

_____

_____

_____

_____

_____

_____

_____

_____

_____

_____

_____

_____

_____

_____

NETTLE PASTA

Put on your gloves, pick a bunch of fresh nettles (the tops are best!), and make this healthy and delicious pasta!

- *Whole (spelt) pasta for 4*
- *1 tbs coconut oil*
- *1 zucchini*
- *4–6 handfuls fresh nettles*
- *2 cups vegetable stock*

- *1 ripe avocado*
- *2 tbs nutritional yeast*
- *Fresh oregano*
- *Pepper*
- *Salt*

Cook the pasta with a little salt in enough boiling water to cover. While the pasta is cooking, melt the coconut oil in a pan. Chop the zucchini and add to the coconut oil. Clean the nettles in cold water and add to the zucchini. Pour in the vegetable stock and stir until the nettles have wilted. Transfer the mixture to a blender. Add the avocado, nutritional yeast and oregano. Blend until smooth. Add pepper and salt to taste. Spoon the pasta and the nettle sauce onto four plates. Add some oregano to garnish.

April 2016

April 2016

				1	2	3
4	5	6	7	8	9	10
11	12	13	14	15	16	17
18	19	20	21	22	23	24
25	26	27	28	29	30	

April 2016

4
MONDAY

5

TUESDAY

6
WEDNESDAY

New Moon 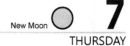 **7**
THURSDAY

8
FRIDAY

9
SATURDAY

10
SUNDAY

April 2016

			1	2	3
4	5	6	7	8	9	10	week 14
11	12	13	14	15	16	17
18	19	20	21	22	23	24
25	26	27	28	29	30

11
MONDAY

12
TUESDAY

13
WEDNESDAY

Sutra IV.10 *tasam anaditvam casiso nityatvat*

First Quarter ☽ **14**
THURSDAY

15
FRIDAY

16
SATURDAY

17
SUNDAY

April 2016

				1	2	3
4	5	6	7	8	9	10
11	12	13	14	15	16	17	week 15
18	19	20	21	22	23	24
25	26	27	28	29	30	

18
MONDAY

19
TUESDAY

20
WEDNESDAY

Sutra IV.11 *hetu phalasrayalambanaih samgrhitatvad esam abhave tadabhavah*

21
THURSDAY

Full Moon ○ **22**
Micro Moon   FRIDAY

23
SATURDAY

24
SUNDAY

April 2016

				1	2	3
4	5	6	7	8	9	10
11	12	13	14	15	16	17
18	19	20	21	22	23	24
25	26	27	28	29	30	

week 16

25
MONDAY

26
TUESDAY

27
WEDNESDAY

Sutra IV.12 *atitanagatam svarupato'sty adhva bhedad dharmanam*

28
THURSDAY

29
FRIDAY

Last Quarter ◖ **30**
SATURDAY

1
SUNDAY

April 2016

				1	2	3
4	5	6	7	8	9	10
11	12	13	14	15	16	17
18	19	20	21	22	23	24
25	26	27	28	29	30	

week 17

Shoelace
Spring - Wood - Anger / Compassion

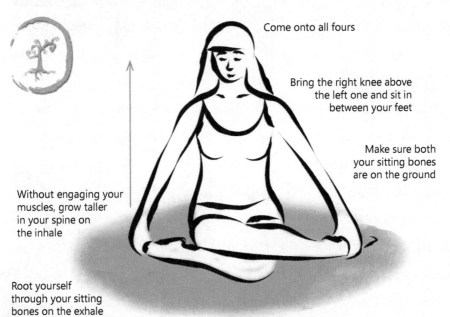

Come onto all fours

Bring the right knee above the left one and sit in between your feet

Make sure both your sitting bones are on the ground

Without engaging your muscles, grow taller in your spine on the inhale

Root yourself through your sitting bones on the exhale

While in the Pose
- Holding time: 3 to 5 minutes on each side.
- Explore suggestions in pp.25-26.

Coming out of the Pose
- Leave the pose slowly and mindfully.
- Exhale and stretch your legs in front of you. Place your hands on the ground behind your hips with your arms extended and lean back, creating a very mild back bend. Repeat on the other side.
- Observe the effects of the pose.

Modifications and Variations
- Sit on a cushion or folded blanket if your hips are tight.
- Stretch the bottom leg if your knees feel challenged.
- Place your hands on the ground next to your hips and rest some weight onto them to make the sensations on the hips and knees less intense.

Taking it Further
- Bend forward, bringing your chest over the top leg, and relax your head completely.
- Bend towards the same side as the top leg and place the forearms on the ground.

Meridian and Associated Emotions

This pose stimulates the Gall Bladder meridian as it flows down through the outer sides of legs, hips and torso, bringing health to this internal organ. The emotions associated with it are Anger (imbalanced) and Compassion (balanced).

Anatomical Benefits

It is a wonderful hip opener.
It decompresses the lower back when bending forward.

Contraindications

Sciatica.
Knee issues.

my notes

Home Practice:
Sequencing Your
Yoga Asanas

By David Lurey

In many aspects of life, the more challenging the task, the greater the reward! Developing an effective home yoga practice is one such concept. The suggestions included in this article will help you to create a personal practice that serves you for each unique moment

When we attend group yoga classes, the teachers create sequences with specific intentions, and as students we can simply follow through the guidance and feel the effects. Most yoga teachers also invite us to "feel into your body" to find the appropriate levels of depth and sensation of each pose. But like a child learning to ride a bicycle with training wheels, once the trainers are taken off, the difficulty increases. When we want to build our own home yoga practice without the teacher's experience and words guiding us, we need to really elevate our level of inner listening in order to create sequences that serve our bodies for each unique day.

To help create a personal yoga practice, it is important to **pay close attention in group classes** to the order of poses our teachers teach and remember them in mind and body. There are fixed sequences, like Sun Salutations, that can be found in a variety of resources for remembering, and then there are the sequences that our favourite teachers teach, making them special to us. Reviewing those unique sequences in our minds immediately after classes and writing them down is a powerful way both to understand how to open the body and to commit the sequences to memory for later recall. Ideally, we can even try them in our bodies again within a day or two, setting them to muscle memory to use later.

In addition to learning how to combine sequences for desired results, it is also important to have a **list of poses and their personal effects**. This is your personal list and will certainly change over time as body, mind and spirit align. An important reflection, when making our list of favourite and challenging poses, is to realise that a body out of balance often craves that which keeps it out of balance. So be sure to include poses on the list that we consciously avoid, as they can bring balance. As long as there is no pain in our body from the poses, including less favourable poses in our home practice will provide a key to continued growth in our personal practice.

To put the poses together in a sequence, there are some **common ideas to consider**.

- What are our intentions for practice (in body, mind and spirit)?

- Do all of the poses work towards or against the intention?
- How do we feel *right now* and what will serve us the most, based on today's life circumstances?

In general, there are groups of poses that target certain body parts, chakras, and even mental states which can be found in books and online. Over time, the common classifications become ingrained into our being and our bodies can work on instinct. This takes time, consistency and patience, but once realised, we can start to practise our own mini home-made sequences, like a laboratory experiment. We can begin with shorter sequences which are easier to keep in memory and build up self-confidence as we *trust ourselves*.

Be aware of the **principle of pose/counter pose** when putting poses together. This simply states that after we stretch or contract a certain part of the body, we do the opposite action to balance it.

If we are sequencing poses to prepare for back-bends, for example, we should avoid forward bending until after we finish all of the back bending. However, after the back bends, a gentle forward bend and/or a twist is important for the counter-balancing.

In addition, if you wish to explore your home practice from an **anatomical perspective**, a general understanding of major muscle groups and joint movements makes sequencing poses like constructing a building. Take each body part separately and explore which muscles need to stretch or strengthen and how the joint will move in peak postures. This way, we build sequences strategically from the foundation up and we can also observe the effects of each stage along the way to determine when to stop or to keep going.

Finally, the Sanskrit word, **tapas**, refers to a positive relationship with discipline; this is one of the more challenging aspects when developing a home practice. Be sure to set aside appropriate time for personal practice, free from distraction, and when finished, take time to feel the effects in order to inform the next

"When we want to build our own home yoga practice without the teacher's experience and words guiding us, we need to really elevate our level of inner listening in order to create sequences that serve our bodies for each unique day."

sequence... that builds the next practice... that informs the next sequence... and on and on.

To learn more about the yogic concept of tapas, please read our article *Light on Tapas* by Clayton Horton (pp.180-182).

my notes

_____

_____

_____

_____

_____

_____

_____

_____

_____

_____

_____

_____

_____

_____

_____

_____

_____

_____

_____

_____

_____

_____

_____

_____

DANDELION: In the Top 10

This sturdy little plant that grows stubbornly in fields, lawns, meadows, or even cracks in the pavement has traditionally been used to treat anaemia, skin problems, blood disorders and many other maladies. But dandelion is also said to rank among the Top 10 green vegetables in overall nutritional value. It is easily available from late spring, when we see its yellow flowers sprouting everywhere, to early autumn, and the whole plant can be eaten: the leaves, the flowers and even the root (roasted as a coffee substitute or cooked as a root veggie). The fresh leaves are a great source of dietary fibre, potassium and magnesium (together they help regulate blood pressure), iron, calcium, zinc, phosphorus and vitamins B and C. Dandelion is one of the highest sources of vitamin A among culinary plants and one of the richest herbal sources of vitamin K.

May 2016

May 2016

						1
2	3	4	5	6	7	8
9	10	11	12	13	14	15
16	17	18	19	20	21	22
23	24	25	26	27	28	29
30	31					

2
MONDAY

3
TUESDAY

4
WEDNESDAY

Sutra IV.13 *te vyakta suksmah gunatmanah*

5
THURSDAY

New Moon ⚪ **6**
FRIDAY

7
SATURDAY

8
SUNDAY

May 2016

						1
2	3	4	5	6	7	8
9	10	11	12	13	14	15
16	17	18	19	20	21	22
23	24	25	26	27	28	29
30	31					

week 18

9
MONDAY

10
TUESDAY

11
WEDNESDAY

12
THURSDAY

First Quarter ◑ # 13
FRIDAY

14
SATURDAY

15
SUNDAY

May 2016

						1
2	3	4	5	6	7	8
9	10	11	12	13	14	15
16	17	18	19	20	21	22
23	24	25	26	27	28	29
30	31					

week 19

16
MONDAY

17
TUESDAY

18
WEDNESDAY

Sutra IV.14 *parinamaikatvad vastu tattvam*

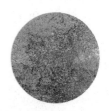

19
THURSDAY

20
FRIDAY

Full Moon ○ **21**
Blue Moon   **SATURDAY**

22
SUNDAY

May 2016

						1
2	3	4	5	6	7	8
9	10	11	12	13	14	15
16	17	18	19	20	21	22
23	24	25	26	27	28	29
30	31					

week 20

23
MONDAY

24
TUESDAY

25
WEDNESDAY

Sutra IV.15 *vastu samye citta bhedat tayor vibhaktah panthah*

26
THURSDAY

27
FRIDAY

28
SATURDAY

Last Quarter ☾ **29**
SUNDAY

May 2016

						1
2	3	4	5	6	7	8
9	10	11	12	13	14	15
16	17	18	19	20	21	22
23	24	25	26	27	28	29	week 21
30	31

Sleeping Swan
Spring - Wood - Anger / Compassion

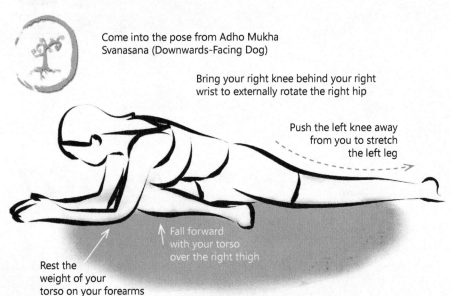

Come into the pose from Adho Mukha Svanasana (Downwards-Facing Dog)

Bring your right knee behind your right wrist to externally rotate the right hip

Push the left knee away from you to stretch the left leg

Fall forward with your torso over the right thigh

Rest the weight of your torso on your forearms

While in the Pose

- Holding time: at least 3 minutes on each side.
- Explore suggestions in pp.25-26.

Coming out of the Pose

- Leave the pose slowly and mindfully.
- Inhale and come up onto your hands to later rest in Balasana (Child's Pose). Repeat on the other side.
- Observe the effects of the pose.

Modifications and Variations

- If you feel too much pressure on the hips, bring the front foot in closer to your pubic bone.
- Play with the position of the legs to make sure your knees are safe.
- Place a cushion or blanket under the front leg's hip to centre yourself if you are leaning to one side.

Taking it Further

- Bring the front foot away from you by opening the knee to the side, and rest your chest on your thigh.
- Tuck in the back foot's toes and lift the back knee off the ground.

Meridian and Associated Emotions

This pose stimulates the Gall Bladder meridian as it flows down through either side of the body along the outer hip, bringing health to this internal organ. The emotions associated with it are Anger (imbalanced) and Compassion (balanced).

Anatomical Benefits

It is a gentle hip opener.
It stretches the IT band (exterior upper leg) and buttock muscles in the front leg.
It stretches the quadriceps and hip flexors in the back leg.

Contraindications

Knee issues.
Hip injuries.

my notes

Summer:
Dancing with Sunlight and Shadow

By Jilly Shipway

The summer solstice in June marks the beginning of the Earth's move towards darkness. It's a perfect time to pause and reflect using the seasonal meditation questions suggested here

The year is a dancing woman, and each season has its own unique dance that presents us with both opportunities and challenges. Becoming familiar with the changing seasons will help us to connect with the earth's cycles and rhythms and notice that we, too, are part of this dance of life. Over time, observing the seasons gives us the wisdom to know when action is required and when it is better just to let things be. We feel more in synch with the flow of life and can relax and enjoy the dance more. Seasonal awareness combines beautifully with yoga and meditation and will enhance both your spiritual practice and your life. One of the best ways to connect with the seasons is to use seasonal meditation questions.

The year can be divided into a light and a dark half. At both the winter and summer solstice there is a shift in the earth's energy. Between the winter solstice in December and the summer solstice in June, the light is expanding; this is the light, yang (sun) half of the year. It may still feel cold and dark at the solstice, but in no time snowdrops and crocuses appear, heralding the start of the growing season. As the sun gets stronger and nature wakes up, the light half of the year supports an outward-looking focus, so it is an auspicious time to get your ideas out into the world.

At the summer solstice, the sun reaches the height of its strength and power and simultaneously there is a shift in the Earth's energy from sun to moon; from fire to water. Slowly the nights begin to lengthen. The dark side of the year supports an inward focus; meditation, reflection and the incubating of ideas for birthing next spring.

Solstice means a stopping or standing still of the sun. Seasonal meditation questions allow us to stop and reflect on how best to use our energy in the coming season.

SEASONAL MEDITATION QUESTIONS can be used:

- During a sitting meditation period
- Whilst relaxing in Savasana (Corpse Pose)
- When you are out on a walk, or during a walking meditation.
- Whilst holding a yoga pose
- As a writing meditation

Choose one or more of the summer solstice meditation questions (below) to work with. Gently repeat the question, maintain-

ing an awareness of your natural breathing, bodily sensations and any thoughts or feelings that arise in response to the question. Let go of hunting for, or pursuing answers to the question. Trust that your subconscious will deliver an answer when the time is right.

- **What have I achieved during the growing season?**
- How will I celebrate my outer achievements?
- Which seeds have failed to germinate and how would I do things differently next time?
- Who has helped me to realise my dreams and how could I thank them?

- **What do I want to incubate during the yin (moon) phase of the year?**
- What do I wish to encourage in my life and what's important to me?
- Which projects and plans do I want to prioritise?
- In order to realise my dreams, what will I need to say "no" to?

- **How do I celebrate the return of the darkness?**
- How do I feel about moving into the dark half of the year?
- How do I balance the light and dark within myself?
- How do I value both my inner and my outer worlds?

"Over time, observing the seasons gives us the wisdom to know when action is required and when it is better just to let things be... Solstice means a stopping or standing still of the sun. Seasonal meditation questions allow us to stop and reflect on how best to use our energy in the coming season."

- **Explore the element of fire:**
- What lights my fire? What is my passion?
- How do I express my creativity and what fuels my creative fire?
- How can I lovingly shine my light out in to the world?

The summer solstice is a fiery and creative time. Bask in the warmth of the sun; celebrate growth and fertility; make love to life itself. At the same time remember to welcome back the darkness which cradles the baby within the womb; nourishes the seed within the soil; rocks you to sleep each night; and gives you the opportunity during the dark half of the year to rest, heal and regenerate.

The year is a dancing woman: allow yourself to be danced.

my notes

DANDELION TAPENADE

The young, fresh leaves and flowers from the dandelion taste the best, but the roots can be eaten as well. For this recipe, use fresh leaves and flowers only. If you soak them in some water with apple cider vinegar for about ten minutes, they will not only be clean and crispy, but will lose some of their bitter taste as well.

- *2 cups green peas*
- *2 cups dandelion, washed*
- *1 avocado, no pit or skin*
- *¼–½ cup water*
- *2 tbs nutritional yeast*

- *2 tbs tahini*
- *½ tsp celtic seasalt*
- *½ tsp paprika powder*
- *½ tsp oregano*

In a food processor or blender, blend all ingredients until a smooth paste forms. Start with the lowest amount of water and add more if needed. You can use more or other spices, according to your taste. Enjoy!

June 2016

June 2016

		1	2	3	4	5
6	7	8	9	10	11	12
13	14	15	16	17	18	19
20	21	22	23	24	25	26
27	28	29	30			

30
MONDAY

31
TUESDAY

1
WEDNESDAY

2
THURSDAY

3
FRIDAY

4
SATURDAY

New Moon ◯ **5**
SUNDAY

June 2016

		1	2	3	4	5	week 22
6	7	8	9	10	11	12	
13	14	15	16	17	18	19	
20	21	22	23	24	25	26	
27	28	29	30				

June 2016

6
MONDAY

7
TUESDAY

8
WEDNESDAY

Sutra IV.16 *na caika citta tantram vastu tadapramanakam tada kim syat*

9
THURSDAY

10
FRIDAY

11
SATURDAY

First Quarter # 12
SUNDAY

June 2016

		1	2	3	4	5
6	7	8	9	10	11	12
13	14	15	16	17	18	19
20	21	22	23	24	25	26
27	28	29	30			

week 23

June 2016

13
MONDAY

14
TUESDAY

15
WEDNESDAY

Sutra IV.17 *taduparagapeksitvac cittasya vastu
jnatajnatam*

16
THURSDAY

17
FRIDAY

18
SATURDAY

19
SUNDAY

June 2016

		1	2	3	4	5
6	7	8	9	10	11	12
13	14	15	16	17	18	19
20	21	22	23	24	25	26
27	28	29	30			

week 24

June 2016

20 ○ Full Moon
MONDAY

21
TUESDAY   Summer Solstice

22
WEDNESDAY

23
THURSDAY

24
FRIDAY

25
SATURDAY

26
SUNDAY

June 2016

		1	2	3	4	5
6	7	8	9	10	11	12
13	14	15	16	17	18	19
20	21	22	23	24	25	26
27	28	29	30			

week 25

June 2016

27 MONDAY
 Last Quarter

28 TUESDAY

29 WEDNESDAY

Sutra IV.18 *sada jnatas citta vrttayas tat prabhoh purusasyaparinamitvat*

30
THURSDAY

1
FRIDAY

2
SATURDAY

3
SUNDAY

June 2016

		1	2	3	4	5
6	7	8	9	10	11	12
13	14	15	16	17	18	19
20	21	22	23	24	25	26
27	28	29	30			

week 26

Seal
Summer - **Fire** - Hate / **Love**

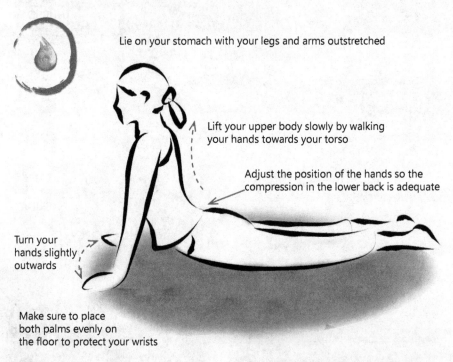

Lie on your stomach with your legs and arms outstretched

Lift your upper body slowly by walking your hands towards your torso

Adjust the position of the hands so the compression in the lower back is adequate

Turn your hands slightly outwards

Make sure to place both palms evenly on the floor to protect your wrists

Coming into the Pose

- Holding time: at least 3 minutes.
- Explore suggestions in pp.25-26.

Coming out of the Pose

- Leave the pose slowly and mindfully.
- Exhale and bend your elbows, lowering yourself to the ground until you are lying on your belly.
- Observe the effects of the pose.

Modifications and Variations

- Lower your torso as much as necessary if the compression in the lumbar area is too intense.
- Slightly bend your elbows if they are hyper-mobile.

Taking it Further

- Turn in your hands so your fingers point towards you to deepen the sensation.
- Allow the head to drop forward or backwards to stretch the neck muscles.

Meridian and Associated Emotions

This pose lengthens the chest away from the abdomen and opens the front of the body, stimulating the Heart meridian as it flows down through the centre of the torso and the inner side of both arms. It can also stimulate the pressure points in the small fingers housing both the Heart and the Small Intestine meridian, bringing health to these complementary internal organs. The emotions associated with them are Hate (imbalanced) and Love (balanced).

Anatomical Benefits

It lengthens the upper torso and opens the chest.
It stimulates the sacro-lumbar arch.
It stimulates the thyroid gland if the head is tilting forward or backwards.

Contraindications

This pose may not be for everyone! If compression in the lower back is too intense, come down into Sphinx Pose, resting on your forearms with your elbows under your shoulders.

my notes

Female Power:
Yoga and the
Divine Feminine

By Nianna Bray

With women being an overwhelming majority in the modern yoga world, a door opens for the Divine Feminine power to manifest in our societies

Women are powerful, yet often don't feel their power. There are many reasons for this, both personal and impersonal. We can look at the implications of patriarchal society, the role of Eve in the Christian creation myth, the unsung heroines left out of textbooks, or our Western history of women not having the right to vote, go to college or own their own property. Looking at history, we can see how far we've come, yet we still have a long way to go. Modern women are ready to step up and out of the past and into a world that honours feminine values and power.

Recently, women have made their way in a man's world, often sacrificing their own feminine essence in the process. To fit in and be seen as equals, women have had to work like men, act like men, and even have sex like men. But we are not men; we are women. While the popularity of yoga has brought the Goddess into the limelight, we are still slightly confused. Women are often objectified or masculinised. There are few role models for feminine power in mainstream outlets. Consequently, women can use this oversight to define what it means to be a woman.

Tantra has re-emerged as a reminder of the great feminine energy called Shakti. Shakti is a Sanskrit word for Divine Feminine Power that is manifest as the universe. In tantric terms, everything is Shakti. Men and women have both masculine and feminine qualities and energy. Humans with more oestrogen are closer to this Divine Feminine Energy. Women have the potential to embody the es-

sence of the Goddess through their female form.

Shakti is not only Divine Feminine Power, but is also sexual energy known as Kundalini. Kundalini is the primordial power within the human body that dwells at the base of our spines and moves up and down the central channel, shushumna nadi, to merge with her beloved Shiva. Shiva is the masculine principle of pure consciousness, transcendent and without form. The two, Shiva and Shakti, become one, and their union is the great love play of Life Itself.

When women come into right relationship with their own sexual energy, they come into contact with their female power. Foolishly, female sexuality has been feared, denied, exploited, usurped, repressed, subjugated, etc. for a very long time. Female sexuality has been misunderstood and hardly investigated by women themselves, but that is changing and very rapidly. Women want to be sexually fluent. There is a movement developing across Europe and the US and into cultures around the world that are deeply steeped in patriarchal male rule.

Now is the time to celebrate female sexuality and truly understand the fullness of its expression, something which benefits both men and women.

"Now is the time to celebrate female sexuality and truly understand the fullness of its expression, something which benefits both men and women. Women's sexuality is powerful, sensual, and imbued with pleasure and ecstasy. Female sexuality, authentically expressed in a woman, empowers all aspects of her life."

Women's sexuality is powerful, sensual, and imbued with pleasure and ecstasy. Female sexuality, authentically expressed in a woman, empowers all aspects of her life. As a woman begins to open to her own orgasmic potential, she turns on an inner switch that lights up her brain. Neurotransmitters send signals of pleasure, joy and contentment throughout her body. Her mind starts to change, as do her behaviours. When a woman feels safe in her body, she opens up to pleasure through sensual pathways; she relaxes and feels secure. This creates the perfect conditions for a woman to awaken and feel empowered in her life and to begin to move in the world from her own centre of strength and confidence. Women who are empowered naturally want to empower others. Women are the cornerstones of their families and that influence spreads out to their communities and beyond.

Yoga has been the perfect breeding ground for the women's empowerment movement to explode. The ratio of women to men who practise yoga makes it glaringly clear that women predominate in the modern yoga world. Yoga has awakened us to our inner power, which is Shakti Herself, and Tantra is the direct realisation path that ushers practitioners, both men and women, to the embodied realisation of Reality through the love play, Lila, of Shiva and Shakti. Through our sadhana, spiritual practice, we have the potential to tap into our Divine Feminine Power and to learn how to live and express it in the world. If you feel a calling to learn, finding a teacher is the first step on the path.

my notes

_____
_____
_____
_____
_____
_____
_____
_____
_____
_____
_____
_____
_____
_____
_____
_____
_____
_____
_____
_____
_____
_____
_____
_____
_____
_____
_____
_____

CHIA SEEDS: Energy and Hydration

These tiny seeds come from the flowers of the *Salvia Hispanica* plant, a member of the mint family. Native to Central America, chia seeds were very important to the Maya and Aztecs due to their capacity to provide sustained energy. Today, we know them as a wonderful source of Omega-3 fatty acids. But that's not all: they are packed with antioxidants, quality protein, and various micronutrients. They contain the amino acid tryptophan that helps regulate appetite and sleep, and they provide calcium, magnesium and phosphorus, thus having a positive effect on bone and oral health. Chia seeds can absorb 10 to 12 times their weight in water; once eaten they form a gel in the stomach that slows the conversion of carbohydrates to sugar, providing energy to mind and body and helping retain hydration during the hottest months of the year.

July 2016

July 2016

					1	2	3
4	5	6	7	8	9	10
11	12	13	14	15	16	17
18	19	20	21	22	23	24
25	26	27	28	29	30	31

July 2016

4 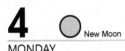 New Moon
MONDAY

5
TUESDAY

6
WEDNESDAY

Sutra IV.19 *na tat svabhasam drsyatvat*

7
THURSDAY

8
FRIDAY

9
SATURDAY

10
SUNDAY

July 2016

			1	2	3
4	5	6	7	8	9	10	week 27
11	12	13	14	15	16	17
18	19	20	21	22	23	24
25	26	27	28	29	30	31

July 2016

11
MONDAY

12 First Quarter
TUESDAY

13
WEDNESDAY

14
THURSDAY

15
FRIDAY

16
SATURDAY

17
SUNDAY

July 2016

				1	2	3
4	5	6	7	8	9	10
11	12	13	14	15	16	17
18	19	20	21	22	23	24
25	26	27	28	29	30	31

week 28

18
MONDAY

19
TUESDAY

20  Full Moon
WEDNESDAY

Sutra IV.20 *eka samaye cobhayanavadharanam*

21
THURSDAY

22
FRIDAY

23
SATURDAY

24
SUNDAY

July 2016

			1	2	3	
4	5	6	7	8	9	10
11	12	13	14	15	16	17
18	19	20	21	22	23	24	week 29
25	26	27	28	29	30	31

25
MONDAY

26
TUESDAY

27  Last Quarter
WEDNESDAY

Sutra IV.21 *cittantara drsye buddhibuddher atiprasangah smrtisamkaras ca*

28
THURSDAY

29
FRIDAY

30
SATURDAY

31
SUNDAY

July 2016

				1	2	3
4	5	6	7	8	9	10
11	12	13	14	15	16	17
18	19	20	21	22	23	24
25	26	27	28	29	30	31

week 30

Shoulder Stretch

Summer – **Fire** – Hate / *Love*

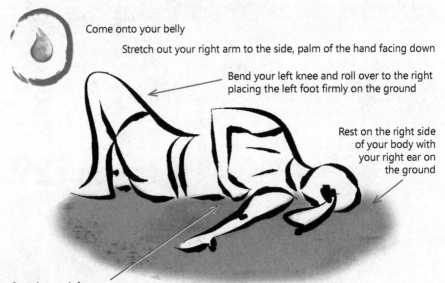

Come onto your belly

Stretch out your right arm to the side, palm of the hand facing down

Bend your left knee and roll over to the right placing the left foot firmly on the ground

Rest on the right side of your body with your right ear on the ground

Stretch your left arm
to the sky and bring it behind your back in a gentle twist

While in the Pose

- Holding time: at least 1 minute on each side.
- Explore suggestions in pp.25-26.

Coming out of the Pose

- Leave the pose slowly and mindfully.
- Exhale and slowly roll back onto your belly, bringing your arms along your body. Repeat on the other side.
- Observe the effects of the pose.

Modifications and Variations

- If the sensation on your shoulders is too intense, come into Wide-Knee Balasana (Child's Pose) and twist to the left, taking the right shoulder under your torso and towards your left knee. Keep your right arm long. Then stretch your left arm to the sky and bring it behind your back in a gentle twist. Rest your cheek on the ground.

Taking it Further

- Try placing more weight on the right shoulder and/or further externally rotate your left hip by pressing your left foot firmly on the ground.

Meridian and Associated Emotions

This pose stimulates the Heart meridian as it flows down through the inner side of both arms, bringing health to this internal organ. The emotions associated with it are Hate (imbalanced) and Love (balanced).

Anatomical Benefits

It stimulates the shoulder joints.
It stretches the adductor muscles.

Contraindications

This pose may not be for everyone!!
Shoulder issues.
Lower back issues.

my notes

_____

_____

_____

_____

_____

_____

_____

_____

_____

_____

_____

_____

Conscious Breathing:
a Master Key for Health

By Alejandra Vidal

Breathing well is a source of our body, gives us mental relaxation

health, as it guarantees greater vitality for clarity, and is a key point for effective

LIVING FAST...
BREATHING FAST

Nowadays, we live immersed in agitated activity which, as a consequence, leads us to do everything quickly. We eat, chat, and even kiss at great speed and, unfortunately, breathing is no exception.

Generally, I dare say that we breathe without rhythm or breaks. In fact, the normal respiratory rate for an adult at rest is eight to 16 breaths per minute, and in profound states of relaxation or meditation, about four times per minute. Several scientific studies have shown that a respiratory rate of eight or less breaths per minute (five seconds inhaling and five seconds exhaling) stimulate the pituitary gland, which is responsible for the regulation of various vital body functions and general well-being. On the other hand, a person who breathes between 20 and 25 times per minute is likely to have, or develop, some sort of nervous or respiratory problem. In addition, we only use 30% of our breathing capacity because, instead of expanding and filling our lungs with air, we tend to breathe superficially. As a consequence, we lack vitality, and we have headaches, anxiety, and stress. But above all, this lack of oxygen leads to the deficient functioning of our entire organism. Although most of us breathe enough not to drown, we do not get the appropriate oxygenation for our bodies.

In view of this, conscious, deep, paused and proper breathing at all times beneficially affects our health, as it facilitates cell and brain oxygenation, regulates heart rate and blood pressure, and favours circulation and digestion. It also acts on our body just as tranquilisers or sedatives do, activating the production of chemicals that produce a feeling of relaxation and tranquillity. In summary, conscious and relaxed breathing can do more than get rid of toxins: it helps us release tension, increases our body awareness, and is a powerful tool for managing our emotions.

LOOK AT A BABY: RELEARN HOW TO BREATHE WELL

Many of the problems that result from the fast-paced life we lead (stress, anxiety, chronic fatigue, depression, muscle tension, insomnia, etc.) could be prevented or mitigated by remembering this master key to health: breathing. Of all the functions of the autonomous system within our bodies (digestion, circulation, etc.) the only one over which we have control is breathing. The best news is that by means of our breathing we can consciously influence our physical and emotional unconscious.

To breathe well, you should do it deeply, subtly and slowly. When inhaling, concentrate on lifting the abdomen and consciously filling the lower, middle and upper parts of the lungs with air. While you hold your breath, feel how the ribs expand on the front and back of your body; the feeling is like slowly inflating a balloon. When you exhale, contract the diaphragm like a bellows and completely rid your lungs of air before breathing again. You only have to look at babies breathing and you will see that their abdomen rises and falls more than their chest and that they do this rhythmically and deeply.

"Conscious, deep, paused and proper breathing at all times beneficially affects our health, as it facilitates cell and brain oxygenation, regulates heart rate and blood pressure, and favours circulation and digestion... It can get rid of more than toxins: it helps us release tension, increases our body awareness and is a great tool for managing our emotions."

gateway to body and mind purification: yogis claim that by creating a habit of proper breathing, the human race would regenerate, causing many diseases to disappear from the face of the earth.

According to yogic philosophy, the invisible vital energy, called prana in Sanskrit, flows throughout the universe and by using breathing techniques we can learn to concentrate, retain, and even guide it within us. Pranayama consists of a series of breathing exercises designed especially to keep the body in a state of vibrant health, calming emotions and generating mental clarity. In other words, this discipline leads us from embracing our breathing to literally transforming ourselves.

CONSCIOUS BREATHING IN YOGA

The benefits of conscious breathing were already known by ancient civilizations. From the beginning, the earliest disciplines, such as yoga, already applied breathing techniques, or pranayama, to purify the organism, stabilize the mind and increase energy levels. Breath control is one of the key elements of yoga, which considers breathing to be the

my notes

_____
_____
_____
_____
_____
_____
_____
_____
_____
_____
_____
_____
_____
_____
_____
_____
_____
_____
_____
_____
_____
_____
_____
_____
_____
_____
_____
_____
_____
_____

MAYAN CHOCOLATE CHIA PUDDING

Perfect for dessert, yet equally awesome for breakfast or lunch. You can make it a day in advance and store it in a fridge, or take all the ingredients with you on a picnic or while travelling and prepare it wherever you are.

- ¼ cup chia seeds
- 1 cup hazelnut-almond milk
- 1 tbs raw cacao
- ¼ tsp cinnamon
- ¼ tsp (or less!) cayenne pepper
- Sweetener to taste

Soak the chia seeds for at least 30 minutes in the hazelnut-almond milk. Transfer the chia mixture to a blender (or just stir the rest of the ingredients in with a spoon or fork), add all other ingredients and blend until smooth. Use as little or as much cayenne pepper as you like. You may want to add a sweetener of your choice to taste. Pour into two bowls, top with cacao nibs and hemp seeds and share with a loved one.

August 2016

August 2016

1	2	3	4	5	6	7
8	9	10	11	12	13	14
15	16	17	18	19	20	21
22	23	24	25	26	27	28
29	30	31				

1
MONDAY

2  New Moon
TUESDAY

3
WEDNESDAY

4
THURSDAY

5
FRIDAY

6
SATURDAY

7
SUNDAY

August 2016

1	2	3	4	5	6	7	week 31
8	9	10	11	12	13	14	
15	16	17	18	19	20	21	
22	23	24	25	26	27	28	
29	30	31					

August 2016

8
MONDAY

9
TUESDAY

10 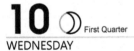 First Quarter
WEDNESDAY

Sutra IV.22 *citer apratisamkramayas tadakarapattau svabuddhisamvedanam*

11
THURSDAY

12
FRIDAY

13
SATURDAY

14
SUNDAY

August 2016

1	2	3	4	5	6	7	
8	9	10	11	12	13	14	week 32
15	16	17	18	19	20	21	
22	23	24	25	26	27	28	
29	30	31					

15
MONDAY

16
TUESDAY

17
WEDNESDAY

Sutra IV.23 *drastr drsyoparaktam cittam sarvartham*

Full Moon ○ **18**
THURSDAY

19
FRIDAY

20
SATURDAY

21
SUNDAY

August 2016

| 1 | 2 | 3 | 4 | 5 | 6 | 7 |
| 8 | 9 | 10 | 11 | 12 | 13 | 14 |
| 15 | 16 | 17 | 18 | 19 | 20 | 21 | week 33
| 22 | 23 | 24 | 25 | 26 | 27 | 28 |
| 29 | 30 | 31 |

22
MONDAY

23
TUESDAY

24
WEDNESDAY

Last Quarter ☾ **25**
THURSDAY

26
FRIDAY

27
SATURDAY

28
SUNDAY

August 2016

1	2	3	4	5	6	7
8	9	10	11	12	13	14
15	16	17	18	19	20	21
22	23	24	25	26	27	28
29	30	31				

week 34

Dragon Flying Low
Late Summer – Earth – Anxiety / Calmness

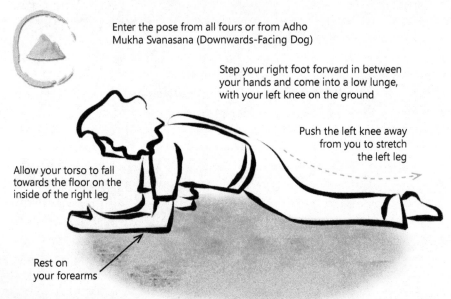

Enter the pose from all fours or from Adho Mukha Svanasana (Downwards-Facing Dog)

Step your right foot forward in between your hands and come into a low lunge, with your left knee on the ground

Push the left knee away from you to stretch the left leg

Allow your torso to fall towards the floor on the inside of the right leg

Rest on your forearms

While in the Pose

- Holding time: at least 3 minutes on each side.
- Explore suggestions in pp.25-26.

Coming out of the Pose

- Leave the pose slowly and mindfully.
- Exhale, gently taking back the right leg and resting in Balasana (Child's Pose). Repeat on the other side.
- Observe the effects of the pose.

Modifications and Variations

- Place a blanket under the back knee or ankle if necessary.
- Placing your hands on the floor, stretch your arms and lift your torso, or even place them on blocks on either side of your front foot.

Taking it Further

- Lift your torso and place your hands on the front leg's thigh, leaning forward to further stretch the back leg hip flexors and quadriceps.
- Enter into a twist, placing the right hand on the right knee, and pushing it to the side while the other hand rests on the floor and the chest rotates to the sky.

Meridian and Associated Emotions

This pose stimulates the Stomach meridian as it flows down through the front of the legs, bringing health to this internal organ. The emotions associated with it are Anxiety (imbalanced) and Calmness (balanced).

Anatomical Benefits

It deeply opens the hips and groins.
It stretches the quadriceps and hip flexors in the back leg.
It stretches the hamstrings in the front leg.

Contraindications

Hip injuries.
Knee or ankle issues.

my notes

Autumn:
Life, Yoga and the Body Clock

By Tina Hedrén

The autumn season is about slowing down, eating and dressing warmly as temperatures fall, as well as evaluating what is important. When it gets darker again and nature draws inwards, we naturally feel less motivated to do a lot. High ideals are good, but life must be practical too!

Most people are aware of the spring equinox and the winter solstice. Living in Sweden, the seasons stand out like different characters that come to pay visits five times per year. The new year begins in the dark, cold winter, with everything resting under the snow. Light returns and sap rises in the trees again with the spring. Summer brings full blossom, long days and midsummer celebration. Nature keeps maturing into the harvest time with its humid nights, when we observe the stars as the days get shorter again.

A different clarity arrives with autumn: the air gets drier and we first see the lack of sunshine in the various colours of the leaves on the trees and bushes. Eventually, the lack of energy will force the leaves to dry out and let go of the branches and nature will stand naked before our eyes. Keywords for the autumn period are discipline, strength, structure, clarity and positive thinking. Reduce unnecessary weight from your shoulders now. To avoid feeling overwhelmed or depressed, let go of old grievances, forgive, and don't live in the past. Get things off your chest; suppressing will deplete your energy.

This is a perfect time to focus on your breath and move with it. Deep breathing helps to let go of habitual tension and release stress. Introduce more pranayama and meditation to shift from an active mind to a more receptive one and the feeling of Oneness.

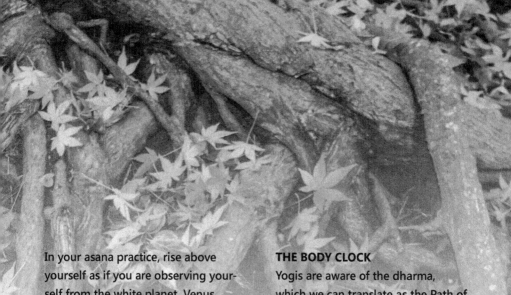

In your asana practice, rise above yourself as if you are observing yourself from the white planet, Venus. How do you shift from one asana to the next? Do you use a lot of effort? Go within and feel your bony structures communicate with each other and then let the muscles take them into action. Strive to make your practice elegant and with beautiful alignment.

During autumn, it is beneficial to build strength from a relaxed body, mind and emotions. As you slow down on the yoga mat and shift from Surya Namaskar (Sun Salutations) to Moon Salutations, you will become aware of stiffness and habitual patterns and you will be able to release them. Though discipline is recommended, always listen; your body knows and feels what it needs, so always allow spontaneous movement.

THE BODY CLOCK

Yogis are aware of the dharma, which we can translate as the Path of Harmony. You may be aware of the Chinese path called the Tao. From Tao, Traditional Chinese Medicine (TCM) evolved. It was early observed that the internal organs work according to a rhythm. We call it the Body Clock.

Traditionally, chi kung practitioners and yogis would do breathing exercises early in the morning, between 3am and 5am. This is the most active time of the lungs, when the energy reaches a peak. Asanas that work to open and close the lungs naturally help with the oxygen exchange. TCM observed that grief weakens the lungs. The energy moves on, reaching a peak at the large intestine between 5am and 7am. It is ideal to eliminate waste in the early morning; TCM also sees this as cleaning out old negativity.

Your lungs and large intestine need extra looking after during the autumn. Other organs need looking after at other seasons.

Energy continues moving to your stomach, where it peaks between 7am and 9am. This is why a good breakfast is recommended. The energy keeps moving around the clock and energy peaks occur at your: spleen, heart, small intestine, bladder and kidneys. As you rest at night, the gallbladder and liver use the energy peak to do their cleaning work between 11pm and 3am.

The Body Clock is a 24-hour clock. At the opposite hours of the peak, an organ is at its weakest time. Most of the time we are not aware of this internal clock, but we certainly feel when we're out of sync, for instance, when we travel over time-zones and get jet-lagged. Working in shifts can also be challenging.

"How do you shift from one asana to the next? Do you use a lot of effort? Go within and feel your bony structures communicate with each other and then let the muscles take them into action. Strive to make your practice elegant and with beautiful alignment."

We would definitely benefit from paying attention to the Body Clock, since modern science relates stress, obesity and insomnia to humans doing things at the wrong hour.

my notes

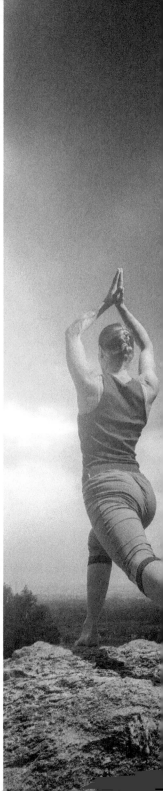

APPLES: A Bite of Freshness

We all have a favourite type of apple among the hundreds of varieties that are cultivated worldwide. The adage "an apple a day keeps the doctor away" is another way of saying that apples are packed with phytonutrients. Biting into an apple is one of those little pleasures of life, and a healthy one at that! Each delicious, crunchy bite acts as a natural mouth freshener that cleans your teeth. Apples contain dietary fibre under the skin that helps prevent the absorption of bad cholesterol. They are rich in vitamin C, a powerful antioxidant that aids the body in fighting infectious agents, which are so common as colder weather sets in. They also provide vitamin B-6, potassium, calcium, iron and zinc. Finally, apples can be the perfect snack, since their low glycemic index makes them release sugar into the bloodstream gradually, providing a sustained source of energy.

September 2016

September 2016

		1	2	3	4
5	6	7	8	9	10	11
12	13	14	15	16	17	18
19	20	21	22	23	24	25
26	27	28	29	30		

29
MONDAY

30
TUESDAY

31
WEDNESDAY

Sutra IV.24 *tad asamkhyeya vasanabhis cittam api*
parartham samhatya karitvat

New Moon ⬤ **1**

Annular Solar Eclipse **THURSDAY**

2
FRIDAY

3
SATURDAY

4
SUNDAY

September 2016

			1	2	3	4	week 35
5	6	7	8	9	10	11
12	13	14	15	16	17	18
19	20	21	22	23	24	25
26	27	28	29	30		

5
MONDAY

6
TUESDAY

7
WEDNESDAY

Sutra IV.25 *visesa darsina atmabhava atmabhava bhavana vinivrttih*

8
THURSDAY

First Quarter ◗ **9**
FRIDAY

10
SATURDAY

11
SUNDAY

September 2016

				1	2	3	4
5	6	7	8	9	10	11	
12	13	14	15	16	17	18	
19	20	21	22	23	24	25	
26	27	28	29	30			

week 36

12
MONDAY

13
TUESDAY

14
WEDNESDAY

15
THURSDAY

Full Moon ○ **16**
Penumbal Lunar Eclipse **FRIDAY**

17
SATURDAY

18
SUNDAY

September 2016

				1	2	3	4
5	6	7	8	9	10	11	
12	13	14	15	16	17	18	week 37
19	20	21	22	23	24	25	
26	27	28	29	30			

19
MONDAY

20
TUESDAY

21
WEDNESDAY

Sutra IV.26 *tadahi viveka nimnam kaivalya pragbharam cittam*

22
Autumn Equinox THURSDAY

Last Quarter ☾ ## 23
FRIDAY

24
SATURDAY

25
SUNDAY

September 2016

			1	2	3	4
5	6	7	8	9	10	11
12	13	14	15	16	17	18
19	20	21	22	23	24	25
26	27	28	29	30		

week 38

26
MONDAY

27
TUESDAY

28
WEDNESDAY

Sutra IV.27 *tacchidresu pratyayantarani samskarebhyah*

29
THURSDAY

30
FRIDAY

New Moon 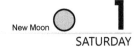 **1**
SATURDAY

2
SUNDAY

September 2016

			1	2	3	4
5	6	7	8	9	10	11
12	13	14	15	16	17	18
19	20	21	22	23	24	25
26	27	28	29	30		

week 39

Half Saddle Variation
Late Summer – Earth – Anxiety / Calmness

Lie on your back in Half Saddle Pose (from Child's Pose, sit up, lean to your right, stretch out your left leg and rest all the way back onto the floor while keeping the right leg folded with the foot near your buttock)

Come up from the back bend, keep your right leg bent back and spread your knees wide open

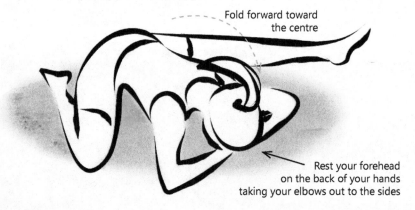

Fold forward toward the centre

Rest your forehead on the back of your hands taking your elbows out to the sides

While in the Pose
- Holding time: at least 3 minutes on each side.
- Explore suggestions in pp.25-26.

Coming out of the Pose
- Leave the pose slowly and mindfully.
- Inhale and slowly come back up to a sitting position. Bring your right leg forward and both legs towards each other. Place your hands on the ground behind your hips with your arms extended and rest back, creating a very mild back bend. Repeat on the other side.
- Observe the effects of the pose.

Modifications and Variations
- Come back up, twist slowly from your hips towards the extended leg and fall forward over it.

Taking it Further
- Come to a sitting position without moving your legs and lean all the way back until you are resting on the floor or on an elevated prop. Make sure your knees are separated to affect the inner legs.

Meridian and Associated Emotions

This pose stimulates the Spleen meridian as it flows up through the inside of the legs, bringing health to this internal organ. The emotions associated with it are Anxiety (imbalanced) and Calmness (balanced).

Anatomical Benefits

It stretches the groins and adductor muscles.
It opens the armpits.

Contraindications

Knee issues.
Hamstring injuries.

my notes

Light on Tapas:
Burning Away the Personal Agenda

By Clayton Horton

When we come across the word tapas, most of us might imagine some delicious appetiser of Spanish cuisine. But to the yoga practitioner, tapas is the sacrifice and the hard work that provides progress and success to any transformational process

In Sanskrit, the word tapas means to burn or glow, referring to a heating process of burning away impurities. In the *Yoga Sutras* of Patanjali, tapas is listed as one of the five niyamas, or observances. The niyamas are the second of the eight limbs of Ashtanga yoga from the Patanjali's *Yoga Sutras*.

In many *Yoga Sutra* commentaries, tapas

is commonly defined as austerity, penance or discipline. Patanjali begins his discussion of sadhana, or spiritual practice, by saying that along with svadyaya (study of the Self) and isvara pranidhana (surrendering to the divine), tapas is a necessary ingredient for any authentic yoga practice (II.1). Without tapas we would never make it onto the mat or meditation pillow and any ordinary effort would not bear much fruit.

By consistent hard work, unhelpful or negative samskaras (habits) and kleshas (root afflictions) are forced to surface in our awareness, be acknowledged, and then discarded, just as a jeweller will heat gold to burn away impurities. Ahimsa (nonviolence) and vairagya (dispassion) have their place in one's life and practice, but we all need to do some authentic personal housecleaning in order to see the brilliance of the jewel of the Self shine forth. To read more about cleansing in relation to yoga practice, read our article *Spring* by Melina Meza (pp.62-64).

Sri K. Pattabhi Jois, in his book, *Yoga Mala*, describes tapas as ob-servances performed to discipline the body and sense organs so that our mind, intellect, ego and faculty of discrimination will become purified, refined and perfected. One simple example of tapas is sitting in a sweltering hot sauna to sweat out toxins. Another example is B.K.S. Iyengar's saying, "the posture begins when you are ready to come out of it." Doing the hard work of staying in the asana, even though our legs are shaking and our breath is becoming unsteady, is what is required for us to develop core strength and stability.

A yogi might spend countless challenging hours in focused meditation, looking deeply at the nature and causes of his suffering. Generally speaking, anything which is difficult, but somehow makes us or our world better, stronger or more mature is regarded as tapas or tapasia.

Swami Satchitananda defines tapas as voluntary suffering for our own purification and development. This intentional suffering is one in which we place ourselves in a situation in which the heat of the moment begins to purify our entire being-physical body, mind, and sense organs included.

On the path to reaching our highest potential, focused intention and action are frequently distracted by six poisons of the individual personality, or desire body. These six poisons are referred to as greed, fear, anger, jealousy, lust and laziness. The honest state of yoga, the union of the individuated Self and the universal Self, occurs when we stop obsessing over ourselves, our story and our desires.

> "In times such as these, when phrases like "my practice" and self-promotional asana selfies posted on Facebook are commonplace, it is important to ask ourselves, or remember, why we are practising yoga in the first place. The greatest happiness is found in helping others."

Sri Anandamurti of the Ananda Marga organisation regards tapas as the hard work or sacrifice that we make for the benefit of others who are in need. This perspective on tapas shines forth as one that promotes cosmic unity and the selfless action known as Karma yoga. Sacrifice here refers to the burning away of our personal desires and agenda to serve the greater whole. In times such as these, when phrases like "my practice" and self-promotional asana selfies posted on Facebook are commonplace, it is important to ask ourselves, or remember, why we are practising yoga in the first place. The greatest happiness is found in helping others.

Embrace tapas by learning to schedule and manage your time. Prioritise your work, play, eating and personal spiritual practice to create a balanced and healthy life of blossoming potential for yourself and others.

To learn more about tapas in the context of a personal practice, please read our article *Home Practice* by David Lurey (pp.96-98).

my notes

RAW APPLE PIE

What is dinner without dessert?! This one is a winner, and you can even eat it during a detox!

- *2½ cups almond flour*
- *1 cup dates, pits removed*
- *¼–½ tsp salt*

Blend all ingredients until a sticky dough forms. Start with the least amount of salt and add more if you wish. If your dough isn't sticky, add more dates. Transfer the dough to a cake pan and press firmly in the pan.

For the filling:

- *3 apples, cores removed*
- *1 cup dates, pits removed and soaked in warm water for 10 minutes*
- *Juice of ½ lemon*
- *1 tsp cinnamon*
- *½ tsp powdered ginger*
- *Pinch of nutmeg (optional)*

Blend all ingredients until a chunky apple mixture appears. Spoon on top of the almond base and place the whole pie in the fridge for at least 15 minutes. Serve with some chopped almonds, raw cacao nibs and a little cinnamon.

October 2016

October 2016

					1	2
3	4	5	6	7	8	9
10	11	12	13	14	15	16
17	18	19	20	21	22	23
24	25	26	27	28	29	30
31						

3
MONDAY

4
TUESDAY

5
WEDNESDAY

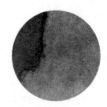

6
THURSDAY

7
FRIDAY

8
SATURDAY

First Quarter ◑ **9**
SUNDAY

October 2016

					1	2
3	4	5	6	7	8	9	week 40
10	11	12	13	14	15	16
17	18	19	20	21	22	23
24	25	26	27	28	29	30
31						

October 2016

10
MONDAY

11
TUESDAY

12
WEDNESDAY

Sutra IV.28 *hanam esam klesavad uktam*

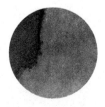

13
THURSDAY

14
FRIDAY

15
SATURDAY

Full Moon 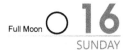 # 16
SUNDAY

October 2016

					1	2
3	4	5	6	7	8	9
10	11	12	13	14	15	16
17	18	19	20	21	22	23
24	25	26	27	28	29	30
31						

week 41

17
MONDAY

18
TUESDAY

19
WEDNESDAY

Sutra IV.29 *prasamkhyane'py akusidasya sarvatha vivekakhyater dharmameghah samadhih*

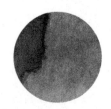

20
THURSDAY

21
FRIDAY

Last Quarter 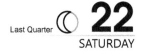 **22**
SATURDAY

23
SUNDAY

October 2016

					1	2
3	4	5	6	7	8	9
10	11	12	13	14	15	16
17	18	19	20	21	22	23
24	25	26	27	28	29	30
31						

week 42

24
MONDAY

25
TUESDAY

26
WEDNESDAY

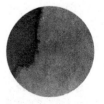

27
THURSDAY

28
FRIDAY

29
SATURDAY

New Moon ⬤ **30**
SUNDAY

October 2016

					1	2
3	4	5	6	7	8	9
10	11	12	13	14	15	16
17	18	19	20	21	22	23
24	25	26	27	28	29	30
31						

week 43

Caterpillar
Autumn – Metal – Sadness / Courage

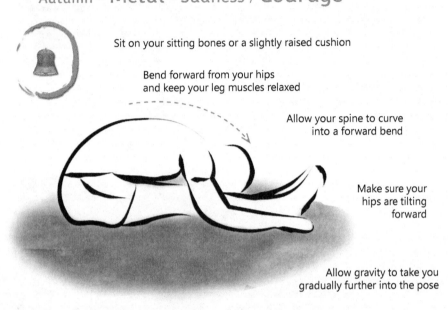

Sit on your sitting bones or a slightly raised cushion

Bend forward from your hips and keep your leg muscles relaxed

Allow your spine to curve into a forward bend

Make sure your hips are tilting forward

Allow gravity to take you gradually further into the pose

While in the Pose
- Holding time: at least 3 minutes.
- Explore suggestions in pp.25-26.

Coming out of the Pose
- Leave the pose slowly and mindfully.
- Inhale and raise your spine slowly, stacking vertebra over vertebra until you are sitting upright. Place your hands on the ground behind your hips with your arms extended and rest back, creating a very mild back bend.
- Observe the effects of the pose.

Modifications and Variations
- Sit with a cushion under your sitting bones if you suffer from sciatica or tight lower back muscles.
- If your hamstrings are tight, bend both knees and place a cushion under them for support.
- Support your neck by resting your head on a cushion or a blanket placed on your legs.

Taking it Further
- Make sure your hips are tilting forward by sitting slightly in front of your sitting bones.
- Open your legs slightly and allow your torso to fall to the ground in between them.

Meridian and Associated Emotions

This pose stimulates the Lung meridian as it flows down through the torso and abdominal region, which are under pressure here, bringing health to these internal organs. The emotions associated with them are Sadness (imbalanced) and Courage (balanced).

Anatomical Benefits

Stretches the ligaments along the back of the spine.

Contraindications

It can aggravate sciatica.

my notes

Ourmala:
Socially Conscious Yoga

By Emily Brett

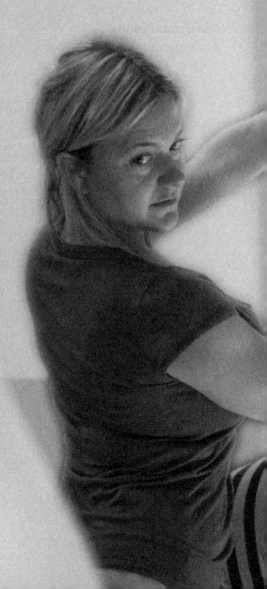

Ourmala is a small London-based charity that makes the benefits of yoga accessible to refugees and asylum-seekers in the city. The core group of students have fled for their lives from their home countries, are unable to live there now for fear of persecution, and are registered with the UK Home Office to seek refuge in the UK

Established in 2011, Ourmala started off working solely with refugee and asylum-seeking women, one of the most vulnerable and under-represented groups in the UK. Many have survived atrocities, such as torture, human trafficking, rape as a tool of war, and other forms of gender-based violence. Ourmala runs on an almost entirely voluntary basis, with most of the funding received spent on refunding the cost of travel for the women to get to yoga, without which most would not be able to attend. They come from all over the world and are referred to Ourmala by organisations, such as Freedom from Torture and British Red Cross Refugee Services.

Now, Ourmala has supported almost 200 women and has waiting lists for its classes. Our patrons include Lindsey Hilsum, the International Editor of the BBC's Channel 4 News.

Yoga is a deeply restorative and healing practice, and at Ourmala, we use our privilege and practice to give access to its benefits to some of those in our community who have suffered most. Yoga is much more than just asana, and Ourmala is part of my personal practice.

Rose*, one of Ourmala's students, has been coming to class for a year and a half. In her twenties now, she was forced into prostitution in her African home country when she was a young teenager. She was raped multiple times and, when she was 16, was trafficked to England. She was referred to Ourmala by an organisation in London that supports survivors of human rights abuse. Rose was very shy at first. It took weeks before she would speak to her fellow yoga students, though she took to yoga practice immediately. She is a lot more confident now, loves a chat with her friends at Ourmala, and is committed to her studies, determined not to let her past dictate her future.

"Yoga gives me hope," says Rose. "It's horrible sometimes—the memories, when I can't sleep, or suddenly in the middle of the day—but yoga helps me leave the past behind. It gives me a peace deep inside and I feel safe, and stronger. Thank you for supporting me and helping me to believe in myself."

Mehret*, a refugee from Eritrea, has been separated from her children and husband since she fled for her life. There is a dictatorship in Eritrea; torture, arbitrary detention, and severe restrictions on freedom of expression are routine, while military conscription is mandatory but has no end date. Mehret has lost two children and her husband to war. She has been with Ourmala for five months and, despite restricted mobility and pain in her body, she is dedicated to her practice.

"I miss my children and husband and I am lonely," says Mehret. "My body hurts. But yoga helps me relax from stress, and sleep. My body pain all goes and I feel more positive. The people are friendly; we are friends. I can touch my toes now. Never before!"

Sarah has been an assistant yoga teacher at Ourmala since 2014 and works closely with the women:

"We women come together as a family every week and the sisterhood we have created shines through in the love and support we offer one another. The environment we foster is nurturing and allows for positive change to take place. I volunteer because I believe it is this kind of collective spirit that we need to harvest and to represent in order to make the world a better place."

To find out more about Ourmala and how you can get involved, visit **www.ourmala.com**. Or donate now at **www.localgiving.com/yoga**

Real names have been changed to protect identity.

"We women come together as a family every week and the sisterhood we have created shines through in the love and support we offer one another. The environment we foster is nurturing and allows for positive change to take place."

Photos by Carl Bigmore

my notes

MISO: The Fermented Superfood

Nothing compares to a piping hot soup during the cold winter months. But if, in addition to warming up, we wish to supply our bodies with a high concentration of nutrients and incredible disease-fighting properties, miso is a great choice. This traditional Asian fermented food is most commonly made from soybeans, sea salt and a yeast mould known as *koji*, often mixed with other grains, such as white or brown rice, barley, or buckwheat and allowed to ferment for anything from several days to several years. Miso is a great source of vitamin B, protein and dietary fibre. Like other fermented and unpasteurised foods, it is an enzyme-rich food and increases the concentration of beneficial probiotic bacteria in the digestive tract, thus aiding digestion, enhancing the body's capacity to extract nutrients from food and, therefore, helping to boost the immune system.

November 2016

November 2016

	1	2	3	4	5	6
7	8	9	10	11	12	13
14	15	16	17	18	19	20
21	22	23	24	25	26	27
28	29	30				

October / November 2016

31
MONDAY

1
TUESDAY

2
WEDNESDAY

Sutra IV.30 *tatah klesa karma nivrttih*

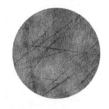

3
THURSDAY

4
FRIDAY

5
SATURDAY

6
SUNDAY

November 2016

	1	2	3	4	5	6	week 44
7	8	9	10	11	12	13	
14	15	16	17	18	19	20	
21	22	23	24	25	26	27	
28	29	30					

7
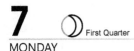 First Quarter
MONDAY

8
TUESDAY

9
WEDNESDAY

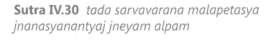

Sutra IV.30 *tada sarvavarana malapetasya
jnanasyanantyaj jneyam alpam*

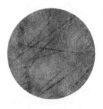

10
THURSDAY

11
FRIDAY

12
SATURDAY

13
SUNDAY

November 2016

1	2	3	4	5	6	
7	8	9	10	11	12	13	week 45
14	15	16	17	18	19	20
21	22	23	24	25	26	27
28	29	30				

November 2016

14
MONDAY

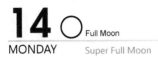 Full Moon

Super Full Moon

15
TUESDAY

16
WEDNESDAY

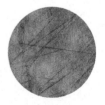

17
THURSDAY

18
FRIDAY

19
SATURDAY

20
SUNDAY

November 2016

	1	2	3	4	5	6
7	8	9	10	11	12	13
14	15	16	17	18	19	20
21	22	23	24	25	26	27
28	29	30				

week 46

November 2016

21
MONDAY 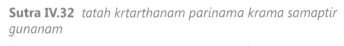 Last Quarter

22
TUESDAY

23
WEDNESDAY

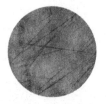

Sutra IV.32 *tatah krtarthanam parinama krama samaptir gunanam*

24
THURSDAY

25
FRIDAY

26
SATURDAY

27
SUNDAY

November 2016

	1	2	3	4	5	6
7	8	9	10	11	12	13
14	15	16	17	18	19	20
21	22	23	24	25	26	27
28	29	30				

week 47

Cat Pulling its Tail
Autumn – Metal – Sadness / Courage

Start by lying on your back

Bring your stretched right leg over your body and towards the left

Lean on the outer side of your left hip in a gentle spinal twist

Bend your left leg behind you and hold your left foot with your right hand

Hold your right foot with your left hand and relax your upper torso to the ground

While in the Pose
- Holding time: at least 1 minute on each side.
- Explore suggestions in pp.25-26.

Coming out of the Pose
- Leave the pose slowly and mindfully.
- Exhale and slowly let go of your feet. Lie flat on your back before bringing your knees to your chest. Circle your knees to one side first and then the other to massage your lumbar area. Repeat on the other side.
- Observe the effects of the pose.

Modifications and Variations
- Prop yourself up on your right upper arm and lean your head on your right hand.

Taking it Further
- Look back over your shoulder and towards your back foot to intensify the twist.
- Pull with your back foot away from your buttock.

Meridian and Associated Emotions

This pose stimulates the Large Intestine meridian as it flows up through the outer side of the arm holding the stretched leg, bringing health to this internal organ. The emotions associated with it are Sadness (imbalanced) and Courage (balanced).

Anatomical Benefits

It gently compresses and stimulates the lumbar area.
It stretches intercostal muscles, quadriceps, hip flexors and pectoral muscles.
It is a good counterpose for intense forward bends.

Contraindications

Lower area issues.

my notes

Winter:
Yantras, Yoga, and You

By Debra Kochanczyk

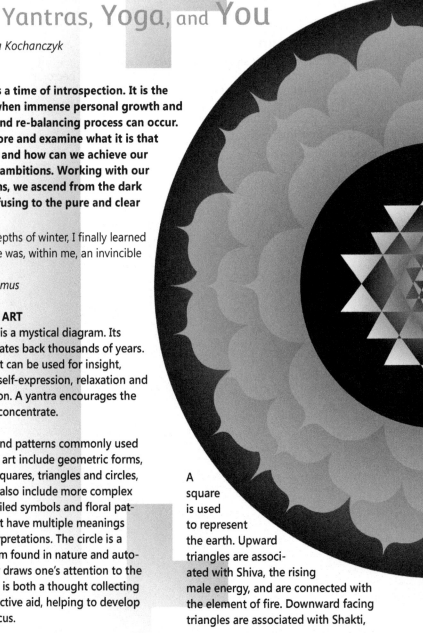

Winter is a time of introspection. It is the season when immense personal growth and a profound re-balancing process can occur. We explore and examine what it is that we want and how can we achieve our goals or ambitions. Working with our intentions, we ascend from the dark and confusing to the pure and clear

"In the depths of winter, I finally learned that there was, within me, an invincible summer."
Albert Camus

YANTRA ART

A yantra is a mystical diagram. Its history dates back thousands of years. Yantra art can be used for insight, healing, self-expression, relaxation and meditation. A yantra encourages the mind to concentrate.

Shapes and patterns commonly used in yantra art include geometric forms, such as squares, triangles and circles, but may also include more complex and detailed symbols and floral patterns that have multiple meanings and interpretations. The circle is a basic form found in nature and automatically draws one's attention to the centre. It is both a thought collecting and reflective aid, helping to develop visual focus.

A square is used to represent the earth. Upward triangles are associated with Shiva, the rising male energy, and are connected with the element of fire. Downward facing triangles are associated with Shakti, the divine and graceful female energy, and are connected with the element of water. The archetypal number 3 is signified by the shape of the triangle and by the Trinity of beginning, middle and end.

petals represents the lotus of creation, while a row of 16 lotus petals represents the lotus of reproductive force.

The colours used in yantra art are also full of meaning and symbolism. The colours of each season have relationships and implications; some colours create an impression of harmony, a message of balance, peace and healing. Other colours clash, suggesting conflict, vitality and disharmony.

The changes of the seasons create different families of colours. Pastel pinks, lavenders and yellows of spring change into rich greens and golds of summer. Autumn brings dark earthy palettes and winter brings extremes of greys, black, and white, suggesting cool winter days, grey skies, long dark nights and the brightness of snow.

YANTRAS AND YOGA

Looking into a yantra stimulates the right hemisphere of the brain, the centre of the emotional, creative, imaginative, intuitive and holistic aspects of our being.

Notably, within the Sri Yantra, so named because it is the mother of all yantras and all other yantras derive from it, the arrangements of shapes and the number of lotus petals are significant. A row of eight lotus

As we begin our yoga practice we can use a yantra as a point of focus for our concentration and our intentions as we develop flexibility and strength in the physical body. During our practice we can use it at the end of each vinyasa or asana, bringing attention back to our intentions. Used at the end of our practice, yantras guide our attention to a point of focus as an aid to meditation, which will enable us to become not only physical, but also spiritual practitioners.

> "The changes of the seasons create different families of colours... winter brings extremes of greys, black, and white, suggesting cool winter days, grey skies, long dark nights and the brightness of snow."

YANTRAS, YOGA, AND YOU

The ancient sages remind us time and time again that the purpose of a yoga practice is to prepare us for meditation. When we have exercised our body, it is then that we can sit in stillness and explore and discover who we really are. When we meditate, we become calm, controlled and balanced.

In the *Yoga Sutras*, Patanjali describes meditation as "a process in which we learn to rest our awareness on a single point."

Harness the power of the yantra to deepen your awareness of your yoga practice, to enrich your meditation practice or just to enjoy its beauty and symmetry.

Allow your own creativity to flow by creating your own yantra. Creating yantras can help to stabilize, integrate and bring order to one's life. The art of creation is always therapeutic and a great way to express your hopes and desires.

Now is the time to prepare for your invincible summer.

Yantra artwork by Debra Kochanczyk

my notes

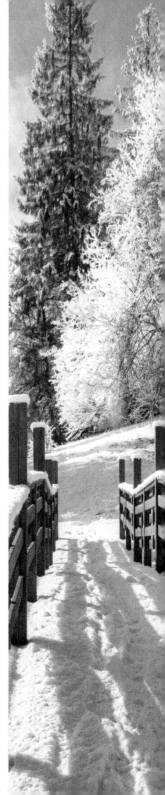

HEALING MISO DAHL

Wash the lentils and soak them overnight (to make them more digestible) together with the kombu and a big splash of apple cider vinegar in plenty of water.

- 4 cups yellow lentils
- 3 stalks of kombu
- Splash of apple cider vinegar
- 2–5 tsp turmeric (fresh or powdered)
- 2–5 tsp ginger (fresh or powdered)
- 1–5 tsp ground black pepper
- 1–3 tsp cardamom powder
- 1–3 tsp cumin powder
- 1–3 tsp coriander powder
- 1–2 tsp cinnamon powder
- 2–4 tbs miso paste (I used Genmai Miso)
- 1 tbs umeboshi paste

The next day, rinse the lentils and kombu. Put in a large pan and add enough water to cover them. Bring to the boil and cook until they are tender. Add the spices according to taste. Remove the pan from the heat. Add the miso paste and umeboshi paste. Use an immersion blender to blend until smooth. Serve and enjoy.

December 2016

December 2016

			1	2	3	4
5	6	7	8	9	10	11
12	13	14	15	16	17	18
19	20	21	22	23	24	25
26	27	28	29	30	31	

28
MONDAY

29
TUESDAY

30 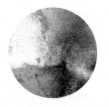 New Moon
WEDNESDAY

Sutra IV.33 *ksana pratiyogi parinamaparanta nirgrahyah kramah*

1
THURSDAY

2
FRIDAY

3
SATURDAY

4
SUNDAY

December 2016

		1	2	3	4	week 48
5	6	7	8	9	10	11
12	13	14	15	16	17	18
19	20	21	22	23	24	25
26	27	28	29	30	31	

5
MONDAY

6
TUESDAY

7
First Quarter
WEDNESDAY

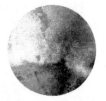

8
THURSDAY

9
FRIDAY

10
SATURDAY

11
SUNDAY

December 2016

			1	2	3	4
5	6	7	8	9	10	11
12	13	14	15	16	17	18
19	20	21	22	23	24	25
26	27	28	29	30	31	

week 49

12
MONDAY

13
TUESDAY

14 ○ Full Moon
WEDNESDAY

Sutra IV.34 *purusarthasunyanam gunanam pratiprasavah kaivalyam svarupa pratistha va citisakter iti*

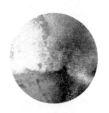

15
THURSDAY

16
FRIDAY

17
SATURDAY

18
SUNDAY

December 2016

			1	2	3	4
5	6	7	8	9	10	11
12	13	14	15	16	17	18
19	20	21	22	23	24	25
26	27	28	29	30	31	

week 50

19
MONDAY

20
TUESDAY

21 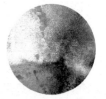 Last Quarter
WEDNESDAY   Winter Solstice

22
THURSDAY

23
FRIDAY

24
SATURDAY

25
SUNDAY

December 2016

			1	2	3	4
5	6	7	8	9	10	11
12	13	14	15	16	17	18
19	20	21	22	23	24	25
26	27	28	29	30	31	

week 51

December 2016

26
MONDAY

27
TUESDAY

28
WEDNESDAY

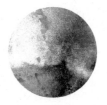

New Moon ○ **29**
THURSDAY

30
FRIDAY

31
SATURDAY

1
SUNDAY

December 2016

			1	2	3	4
5	6	7	8	9	10	11
12	13	14	15	16	17	18
19	20	21	22	23	24	25
26	27	28	29	30	31	

week 52

Dangling
Winter - Water - Fear / Wisdom

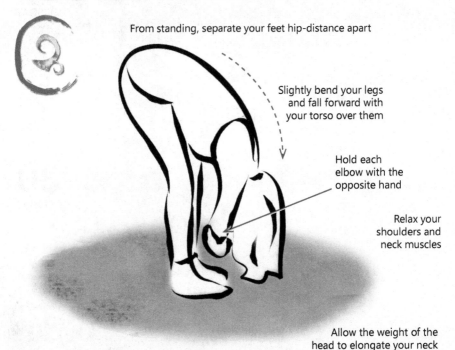

From standing, separate your feet hip-distance apart

Slightly bend your legs and fall forward with your torso over them

Hold each elbow with the opposite hand

Relax your shoulders and neck muscles

Allow the weight of the head to elongate your neck

While in the Pose
- Holding time: at least 2 minutes.
- Explore suggestions in pp.25-26.

Coming out of the Pose
- Leave the pose slowly and mindfully.
- Exhale and lower yourself into a squat. Then sit and do a mild back bend such as Ardha Purvottanasana (Reversed Table Top).
- Observe the effects of the pose.

Modifications and Variations
- If you have any lower back issues, bend your knees as much as necessary, or rest your elbows on your thighs.
- Rest your elbows on a table or the back of a chair if your back doesn't allow for a lot of bending.

Taking it Further
- If you are very flexible, hold your wrists (or elbows) behind your legs instead of in front of them.
- Do the pose with your back against a wall to go deeper into the forward bend.

Meridian and Associated Emotions

This pose stimulates the Urinary Bladder meridian as it flows through either side of the spine and down into the back of the legs, bringing health to this internal organ. The emotions associated with it are Fear (imbalanced) and Wisdom (balanced).

Anatomical Benefits

It gently stretches the lumbar and sacral area.
It warms up hamstrings and quadriceps.

Contraindications

High blood pressure and glaucoma.
Lower back issues.

my notes

Yoga Festivals

AND CELEBRATIONS AROUND THE GLOBE

Curated by Michelle Taffe from theglobalyogi.com.
For up to date information on all of these events check:
http://www.theglobalyogi.com/events/category/festivals-conferences

JANUARY

Yoga Journal Conference
(San Francisco, USA)
5 days of yoga with classes in all
styles and for all levels.
www.yjevents.com/sf

Evolve Yoga and Wellness Festival
(Various locations, Australia)
1 day for the coming together of
the Southern Hemisphere yoga and
wellness community in Byron Bay,
Melbourne and Sydney.
www.evolveyogafestival.com.au

Kundalini Yoga Festival
(San Esteban, Chile)
7 days of Kundalini yoga practice,
expanding on the teachings of Yogi

Bhajan in the mighty Chilean Andes.
www.festivalkundalini.com

Austria Yoga Conference
(Wels, Austria)
3 days of a wonderful range of different yoga styles from international
teachers in the small town of Wels.
www.yoga-conference.at

FEBRUARY

Denver Chant Fest
(Denver, USA)
3 days of chanting and yoga, bringing
North America's top bhakti musicians,
beloved sound-smiths and an array of
local live musicians and DJs to Colorado.
http://denverchantfest.com/

Yogafest
(Dubai, UAE)
3 days of yoga in a tranquil outdoor setting in Dubai. This is a free, sustainable community event supported by volunteers and sponsorships.
www.yogafest.me

Texas Yoga Conference
(Houston, USA)
3 days of yoga, motivational speakers and fun musical evening concerts in Houston.
http://texasyogaconference.com/

Olis Festival
(Milan, Italy)
2 days dedicated to the innate wellness of the body, mind and spirit in Milan.
http://www.olisfestival.it

MARCH

International Yoga Festival
(Rishikesh, India)
7 days on the banks of the sacred river Ganga; a week-long celebration of yoga and one of the world's largest yoga events. Learn from the best of India's spiritual leaders.
www.internationalyogafestival.com

Canon Beach Yoga Festival
(Cannon Beach, USA)
3 days of yoga, art, health, wellness treatments, spa and fun on the Pacific Northwest coast of the US.
www.cannonbeachyogafestival.com

Yoga Australia Conference
(Sydney, Australia)
2 days of yoga and discussion in Sydney providing participants with a chance to learn from some of the most experienced and innovative teachers in Australia.
www.yogaaustraliaconference.org.au

Byron Spirit Festival
(Byron Bay, Australia)
3 days of inspirational yoga, music, tantra and dance in beautiful Mullumbimby, Byron Shire.
www.spiritfestival.com.au

Spirit Fest
(Cape Town, South Africa)
3 days in the crisp mountain air practising yoga, meditation and a healthy life, with the core mission of creating community around mindful living in Cape Town.
www.spiritfest.co.za

Yoga Art Festival Mexico
(Amecameca, Mexico)
6 days of awakening, exploring the potential of human creativity and yoga in the foothills of a sacred volcano.
www.yogaartfestival.com

Bali Spirit Festival
(Ubud, Indonesia)
6 days of yoga workshops, concerts, healing and community, magnified by the magical spirit of the island of Bali.
www.balispiritfestival.com

APRIL

Yoga Journal Conference
(New York, USA)
5 days of yoga with classes in all styles and for all levels.
www.yjevents.com/ny/

MAY

Shakti Fest
(Joshua Tree, USA)
3 days dedicated the devotional path and the Divine Feminine that dwells within all of us with yoga, kirtan and meditation.
http://shaktifest.bhaktifest.com/

Yoga and Holistic Europe Meeting
(Merano, Italy)
2 days over a weekend completely dedicated to finding harmony through yoga practice in the South Tyrol.
www.yogameeting.org

Yoga Festival
(Catania, Italy)
3 days completely dedicated to living and practising harmony through yoga on the beautiful and bountiful island of Sicily.
www.yogafestival.it

The Great British Kundalini Yoga Festival
(Berkshire, England)
5 days of yoga in a friendly, nurturing environment of joy, devotion and service to all beings, rooted in the Kundalini yoga teachings of Yogi Bhajan.
www.kundaliniyogafestival.org.uk

Midsummer Festival of Yoga
(Dorset, England)
4 days of 'celebrating diversity in yoga' with workshops, discussions, music, dance and more in the English countryside.
www.yogafestival.org.uk

German Yoga Conference
(Cologne, Germany)
4 days to 'find freedom' in Cologne, at one of the most established yoga gatherings in Europe.
www.yogaconference.de

JUNE

Colourfest
(Dorset, England)
4 days of celebrating life through the 'colours' of yoga, music and dance. Colourfest offers a wonderful space in which to meet, play, connect and inspire.
http://colourfest.co.uk/

Hanuman Festival
(Boulder, USA)
4 days of community-orientated, world-class yoga and mind-blowing music set at the foot of Colorado's Rocky Mountains.
www.hanumanfestival.com

Bhakti Yoga Summer
(Chiemsee, Germany)
4 days of love, yoga and music in the Bavarian countryside. Join in celebrating the 'flowering of the heart'.
http://bhaktiyogasummer.com

Evolution Asia Yoga Conference
(Hong Kong, China)
4 days of yoga in Hong Kong at Asia's largest annual yoga and wellness conference serving the growing interest in yoga in the region.
www.asiayogaconference.com

Solstice Yoga Festival
(Latvia)
3 days celebrating the European summer solstice (near Riga). With yoga, flowers, special foods and singing to celebrate the season in this thousand year old Latvian tradition.
www.solsticeyogafestival.com

Dutch Yoga Festival
(Terschelling, The Netherlands)
3 days immersed in yoga on a Dutch island, enjoying beaches, camping, lake swimming, cycling and more.
www.yogafestival.info

Bhakti Fest Midwest
(Madison, USA)
3 days celebrating devotion through music, chanting, yoga, meditation and community in Wisconsin.
http://midwest.bhaktifest.com/

JULY

Wanderlust Festival
(Aspen and the Squaw Valley, USA)
4 days to share yoga in rural Colorado or California together with great yoga teachers, musicians, artists and performers.
www.wanderlustfestival.com

Barcelona Yoga Conference
(Barcelona, Spain)
5 days of inspiration in Barcelona with a team of renowned and dedicated teachers offering their personal vision of the ancient yogic wisdom.
www.barcelonayogaconference.cat

Berlin Yoga Festival
(Berlin, Germany)
4 days to cherish 'every breath you take' in yoga, outdoors at the Kladow Kultural Park.
www.yogafestival.de

Bliss Beat Festival
(Sezzadio, Italy)
4 days in the Italian countryside sharing the magic of yoga and devotional kirtan.
www.blissbeatfestival.com

Telluride Yoga Festival Midwest
(Telluride, USA)
4 days of yoga, hiking, social events, music, meditations, SUP yoga, Ayur-vedic dinners, all-day workshops and more in this picturesque valley hidden in the mountains of Colorado.
www.tellurideyogafestival.com

Ängsbacka Yoga Festival
(Molkom, Sweden)
7 days in the Nordic countryside focusing on Ahimsa, bringing peace and freedom to yourself and the world, with yoga enthusiasts of all levels and traditions.
http://en.angsbacka.se/

AUGUST

European Yoga Festival
(Fondjouan, France)
9 days of Kundalini yoga following the teachings of Yogi Bhajan, in a fairytale-like French chateau in a forest. Swim in one of two lakes on the property in between yoga sessions!
www.3ho-kundalini-yoga.eu

Finger Lakes Yoga Festival
(Ithaca, USA)
4 days to celebrate yoga, music and art in the stunning countryside of Ithaca, in New York State. This is a rustic, community-orientated festival.
www.fingerlakesyogafestival.org

Wake Up Festival
(Estes Park, USA)
5 days to 'wake up' in the mountains of Colorado. This festival is designed to engage, inspire, connect and awaken body and soul through talks, ritual and celebration.
http://wakeupfestival.com/

NavaNadi Yoga Festival
(Torhout, Belgium)
3 days of yoga, music and meditation in the Belgian countryside. A smaller, community-based festival.
www.navanadifestival.com

SEPTEMBER

Bhakti Fest West
(Joshua Tree, USA)
4 days celebrating devotion through music, chanting, yoga, meditation and community in California.
http://west.bhaktifest.com/

Yoga Festival
(Rome, Italy)
3 days over a weekend completely dedicated to finding harmony through yoga practice in Rome.
www.yogafestival.it

Geneva Yoga and Music Festival
(Geneva, Switzerland)
5 days of yoga, kirtan, acrobatics, massage and more with a focus on creating peace in the heart of a multicultural community.
www.genevayogamusicfestival.ch

OCTOBER

Yoga Festival
(Milan, Italy)
3 days over a weekend completely dedicated to finding harmony through yoga practice in Milan.
www.yogafestival.it

Kundalini Yoga Asia Festival
(Thailand)
5 days dedicated to serve, inspire and empower humanity to be healthy, happy and whole through the teachings of Kundalini yoga in Thailand.
www.kundaliniyogaasia.org

Ojai Yoga Crib
(Ojai Valley, USA)
4 days of yoga in the Ojai Valley in California, a magical spot long regarded as a place for spiritual pilgrimage. This is a rich spiritual experience with a focus on following the guidance of love.
www.lulubandhas.com/yoga/crib

NOVEMBER

Namaste Festival
(Jakarta, Indonesia)
3 days bringing yoga, healing and related disciplines to Jakarta with the goal of making the Indonesian capital an international well-being destination.
www.namastefestival.com

Dubai Yoga and Music Festival
(Dubai, UAE)
3 days of yoga, music and meditation in the Middle East; 'Shakti in the dunes – fruits of the desert'!
www.dubaiyogafest.com

DECEMBER

Uplift Festival
(Byron Bay, Australia)
4 days to listen to global pioneers from all walks of life come together to share their gifts. Discover the limitless possibilities that emerge when we unify our visions for the greater good of all.
www.upliftfestival.com

Who Contributed
YOGAGENDA 2016

This short presentation is always the very last thing I write for Yogagenda. When all the contents are ready and the graphic design is almost finished, I sit down to put together these few lines. And all I feel there is left to say is thank you.

Thank you to all the contributors, for whom a short biographical note and links to their wonderful yoga work can be found below; it is always a pleasure and a privilege to be able to work with them.

Thank you to you, our reader, who encourages us to keep publishing via emails with feedback all throughout the year. I'm grateful (and thrilled!) to be able to share with you again a new edition of Yogagenda.

Elena

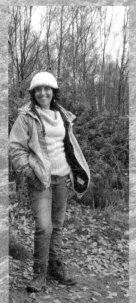

Elena Sepúlveda
(Superfoods: Natural Choices for Superhealth; Asana Overview: Yin Asanas for Self-Transformation; Asana Pages)

As founder, publisher and editor of *Yogagenda*, Elena is the beating heart of this project that brings together her love for yoga and her passion for publishing. She is a yoga teacher (Vinyasa and Yin) and a body worker (Chavutti Thirumal), but also a freelance writer and translator. Her aim is to blend both facets creatively and to find enjoyable and beneficial ways of sharing the results.

Seed-Joy.com

YogagendaS.com

Nianna Bray
(Female Power: Yoga and the Divine Feminine)
Nianna Bray is a tantric yogini who travels the world teaching the wisdom of embodiment. She lights a fire in the hearts of her students and gives them the tools to tend the flame. She is honoured to contribute to this edition of *Yogagenda* and looks forward to meeting you along the path.
NiannaBray.com
AwayInward.com

Emily Brett
(Ourmala: Socially Conscious Yoga)
Emily Brett is a yoga teacher and founder of Ourmala, a small UK-based charity that helps the refugee and asylum-seeking community in London. She specialises in teaching women who have experienced atrocities such as torture, sexual violence in conflict, human trafficking and FGM (female genital mutilation).
OurMala.com
LocalGiving.com/yoga

Tina Hedrén
(Autumn: Life, Yoga and the Body Clock)
Tina is based in Sweden and teaches Seasonal Hatha, a type of yoga that flows in harmony with the seasons. She is a Yoga Alliance affiliate and offers trainings, workshops and retreats for the Scandinavians. Together with her colleague, Sue Wood, she has created two unique *Body Clock* DVDs as a medium for sharing more information.
SeasonalYoga.se

Clayton Horton
(Light on Tapas: Burning Away the Personal Agenda)
Clayton Horton is the director of Greenpath Yoga. He has been a student of yoga since 1988. Clayton has studied with both masters, Sri K. Pattabhi Jois and the Greensufi, for a period of over 14 years. His practice and teachings are rooted in the Ashtanga Vinyasa tradition and daily meditation.
GreenPathYoga.org
AshtangaYoga108.com

Debra Kochanczyk
(Winter: Yantras, Yoga and You)
Debra is a co-founder of OmAge Yoga, Honoring the Journey of Life and the director of OmAge International Yoga Teacher Training School. She lives in Abu Dhabi and is a passionate and internationally renowned yoga teacher and a harmony enthusiast, who discovered the ancient yantra art form through yoga.
OmAgeYoga.com

David Lurey
(Home Practice: Sequencing Your Yoga Asanas)
Radiating enthusiasm and love, David

Lurey teaches Vinyasa yoga for a connection to the self; Acroyoga for connecting to other humans; Green yoga as a way to connect more deeply with the planet and cosmos and Bhakti yoga for divine connections. It is his passion to create intelligent and inspiring yoga classes and workshops, which touch body, mind and spirit at every chance.
FindBalance.net
DavidLurey.bandcamp.com

Josep Macizo
(Web design for www.YogagendaS.com and Yogagenda's graphic design)
Josep is a very precise and versatile web and graphic designer focused on producing sites and publications that reflect his client's needs and identity, may it be a multilayered on-line shop, a complex site with the organic look and function of a paper notebook... or a *Yogagenda*! Technology aside, he also studied fine arts, loves drawing in all its forms and is happy as a child with a pencil in his hands.
JMacizo.com

Melina Meza
(Spring: an Ayurvedic Perspective)
Melina has been exploring the art and science of yoga and nutrition for over 20 years. She combines her knowledge of Hatha yoga, Ayurveda, wholefoods nutrition and healthy lifestyle promotion into a unique style called Seasonal Vinyasa. Meza

is the author of the *Art of Sequencing books* and the DVD, *Yoga for the Seasons – Fall Vinyasa.*
MelinaMeza.com

Swami Saradananda
(Mudras: an Introduction)
Swami Saradananda is an internationally renowned yoga-meditation teacher, who inspires you to want to practice. She is the author of a number of books, including *Chakra Meditation, Power of Breath, Yoga Mind and Body, Relax and Unwind with Yoga, Essential Guide to Chakras* and *Mudras for Modern Life.* After working with Sivananda Yoga Centres for many years, she undertook intensive personal practice in the Himalayas. Now based in London, she teaches workshops and courses worldwide.
FlyingMountainYoga.org

Jilly Shipway
(Summer: Dancing with Sunlight and Shadow)
Jilly is an experienced BWY teacher who offers yoga and mindfulness classes and workshops in Shropshire, U.K. Over the past ten years, she has explored how yoga can be combined with an awareness of the seasons and the earth's cycles, in a way that helps us to embody our spirituality in our everyday lives.
YogaCycles.com
YogaSeasonal.weebly.com

Michelle Taffe
(Yoga Festivals and Celebrations)
Michelle Taffe is the founder of The Global Yogi, a website and online community that connects yogis with teachers, studios, retreat centres, and yoga and spirit events worldwide. The Global Yogi is updated regularly with articles about yoga, personal growth and spiritual development. Michelle is based in Australia and travels regularly, reporting on yoga and the spiritual path worldwide.
TheGlobalYogi.com

Denise Ullmann
(Yogagenda's logo; Illustrations for Asana Pages)
Denise was born in Buenos Aires and she practises yoga, Acroyoga, and dancing, but above all, she has painted for as long as she can remember. Since studying arts, she has worked on a variety of projects, such as illustrating logos for festivals, postcards, CD covers, and stories. She has also edited her own first illustrated book, *Asai Va.*
AbriendoUnMundo.blogspot.com

Irina Verwer
(Recipes for Superfoods)
Irina is intensely grateful for all of life's gifts, including the opportunity to share her love for yoga and food through teaching—online, in her yoga studio or around the globe. She also loves to write about her favour-
ite topics. As a yogic foodie, Irina is constantly inventing new recipes; she wrote the yogic cookbook *Kopstand in de Keuken (Headstand in the Kitchen)*; and she writes blogs about yoga, health and food.
IrinaVerwer.com

Alejandra Vidal
(Conscious Breathing: a Master Key for Health)
Alejandra is a journalist, coach and certified yoga teacher. She currently works on different editorial and journalistic projects, while teaching yoga classes, workshops and seminars in Barcelona. For four years now, Alejandra has been patiently nurturing a personal project that combines the corporative and the spiritual, Corporate Yoga, through which she offers yoga classes and relaxation and meditation techniques adapted to the needs of people in business.
Corporate-Yoga.es

Mirjam Wagner
(Beyond the Mat: Buddhism, Mindful Awareness and Meditation)
Mirjam focuses on transmitting the wisdom of the human body and its close connection to emotional experiences in a simple, transparent and very effective way. Sarah Power is her most significant influence for Buddhism, mindful awareness and daily meditation practice.
YogaTherapyMallorca.com

JOURNAL

Sanskrit
GLOSSARY

Adi Mudra: a hand gesture or seal done by making fists with your thumbs inside your fingers.

Ahimsa: non-violence; one of the five yamas within Patanjali's eight-limbed path of yoga.

Asana: pose or posture; third stage in Patanjali's eight-limbed path of yoga.

Ayurveda: "the Knowledge of Life", a traditional Indian medicine system that uses the principles of nature to maintain health and balance.

Brahma Mudra: a hand gesture or seal done by placing your fists on either side of your navel.

Chakras: subtle energy centres at the hub of a person's being.

Chin Mudra: a hand gesture or seal done by joining the tips of your thumbs and index fingers.

Chinmaya Mudra: a hand gesture or seal done by keeping your thumbs and index fingers joined while bending the middle, ring and little fingers on each hand until they touch their respective palms.

Dharma: virtue or true way of life. It can also be translated as "the Path of Harmony".

Dosha: different constitution types according to Ayurveda; there are three doshas: vata, pitta, kapha.

Duhkha: a Buddhist term commonly translated as suffering, unsatisfactoriness, or unease.

Isvara Pranidhana: surrendering to a principle larger than self; one of the five niyamas in Patanjali's eight-limbed path of yoga.

Kapha dosha: one of the three Ayurvedic types, ruled by earth/water.

Karma yoga: the path of selfless service; one of the four main margas or yoga paths mentioned in the Bhagavad Gita as ways to reach liberation.

Kleshas: root aflictions. According to the *Yoga Sutras*, there are five reasons or kleshas which are the cause of our suffering.

Kundalini: dormant energy located at the base of the spine and often represented as a coiled snake. Also a school or style of yoga.

Lila: the divine play, the play of creation, destruction, and re-creation, the folding and unfolding of the cosmos. It also means love.

Mantra: sacred sound.

Mudra: lit. seal; precise hand and finger gestures used to channel subtle energy or prana.

Nadis: subtle energy paths.

Nadānusandhana: a four-part series of hand seals or mudras practised alongside the different sounds that make up the mantra OM.

Namaste: a spoken greeting or salutation commonly used in India and among yogis everywhere.

Niyama: five self-observances when relating to the inner world; second stage in Patanjali's eight-limbed path of yoga.

OM: the sound of the infinite, representing all that was, is and shall be.

Patanjali: the compiler of the *Yoga Sutras*.

Pitta dosha: one of the three Ayurvedic types, ruled by fire/water.

Prana: subtle or vital energy.

Pranayama: breathing technique; fourth stage in Patanjali's eight-limbed path of yoga.

Sadhana: practice.

Samskara: habit; a repetitive way of thinking that defines behaviour and personality.

Shakti: the feminine, active, immanent, temporal principle.

Shiva: the Hindu god of destruction and one of the Trimurti, the others being Vishnu and Brahma. Also, the masculine, passive, transcendent, eternal principle.

Sushuma: central energy channel

or nadi through which the kundalini energy rises.

Sthira: steadiness, stillness; one of the two qualities of asana mentioned in Patanjali's *Yoga Sutras*.

Sukha: ease, comfort; one of the two qualities of asana mentioned in Patanjali's *Yoga Sutras*.

Sutras: lit. thread; aphorisms about the yogic lifestyle compiled by the sage Patanjali.

Svadyaya: the study of yoga texts; one of the five niyamas in Patanjali's eight-limbed path of yoga.

Tantra: a technique to grow beyond physical limitations.

Tapas: discipline; one of the five niyamas in Patanjali's eight-limbed path of yoga.

Vairagya: dispassion or detachment.

Vata dosha: one of the three Ayurvedic types, ruled by air/space.

Vedas: Hindu sacred scriptures from which all yoga originates.

Vinyasa: fluid sequence of asanas synchronised with breathing.

Yantra: a diagram used as a meditative tool.

Yoga: lit. to yoke or unite; spiritual practice concerned with union.

Yoga sutras: guidelines compiled by Patanjali for those aspiring to higher states of consciousness and liberation.

Yogi/yogini: a person who practices yoga.

JOURNAL

Asana
INDEX

Yoga
SESSION PLANNER

Date/Time: Duration:

Anatomical Focus:

Broader Theme:

Mantra:

Pranayama:

Warm-Ups:

Surya Namaskar:

asanas

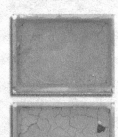

asanas

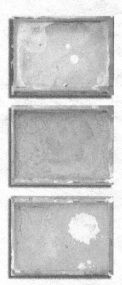

Notes/Insights:

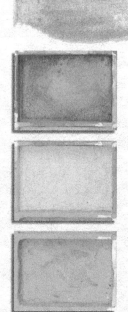

asanas

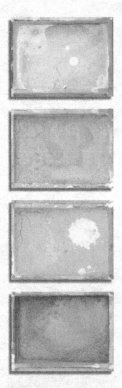

Notes/Insights:

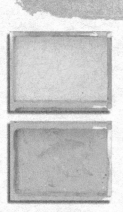

asanas

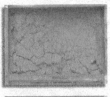

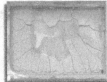

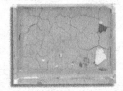

Music:

Relaxation:

Closing/Announcements:

For next session:

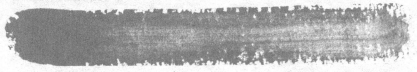

JOURNAL

JOURNAL

JOURNAL

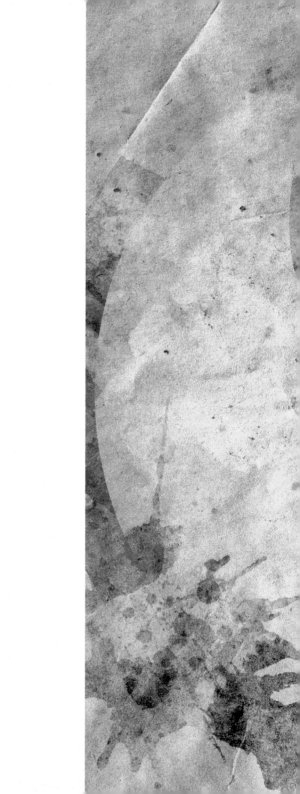

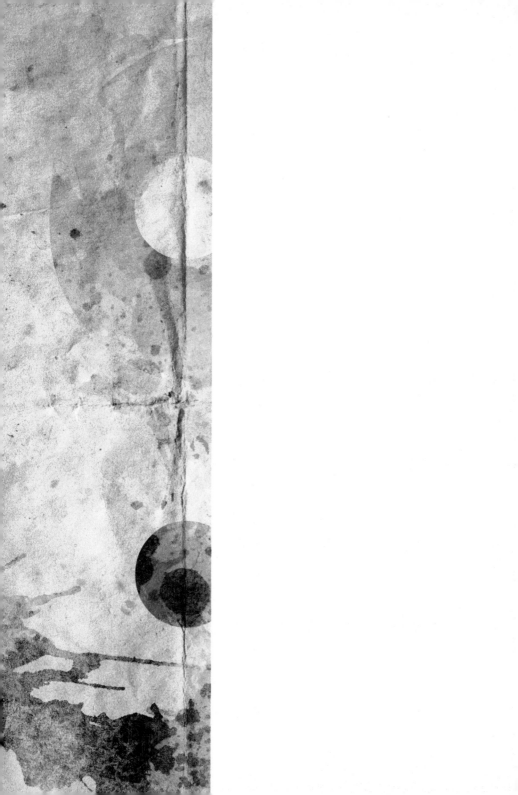

JOURNAL

JOURNAL

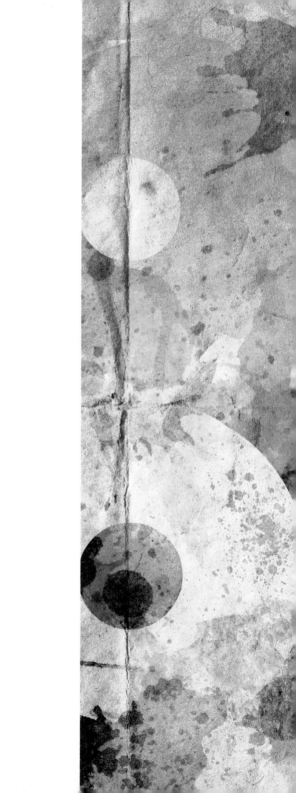

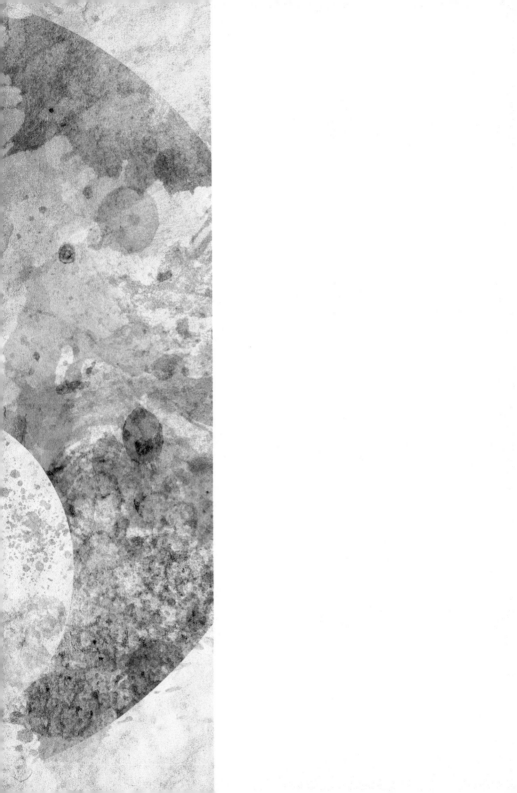

JOURNAL

JOURNAL

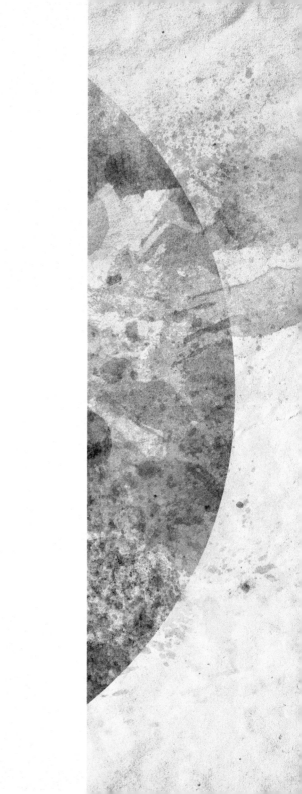

JOURNAL

CPSIA information can be obtained
at www.ICGtesting.com
Printed in the USA
LVOW02s2044301115

464709LV00016B/50/P